PUBLIC HEALTH IN THE 21ST CENTURY

MRSA (METHICILLIN RESISTANT *STAPHYLOCOCCUS AUREUS*) INFECTIONS AND TREATMENT

PUBLIC HEALTH IN THE 21ST CENTURY

MRSA (Methicillin Resistant Staphylococcus aureus)
Infections and Treatment
Manal M. Baddour
2010. ISBN: 978-1-61668-038-1
2010. ISBN: 978-1-61668-450-1 (E-book)

Influenza Pandemic - Preparedness and Response To A Health
Disaster
Emma S. Brouwer (Editor)
2010. ISBN: 978-1-60692-953-7
2010. ISBN: 978-1-61728-041-2 (E-book)

Biofunctional Scaffolds for Spinal Cord Regeneration
Jerani T. S. Pettikiriarachchi, Malcolm K. Horne,
John S. Forsythe and David R. Nisbet
2010. ISBN: 978-1-61668-757-1
2010. ISBN: 978-1-61728-256-0 (E-book)

Infectious Disease Modelling Research Progress
Jean Michel Tchuenche and C. Chiyaka (Editors)
2010. ISBN: 978-1-60741-347-9

Home Fire Safety: Preventive Measures and Issues
Cornelio Moretti (Editor)
2009. ISBN: 978-1-60741-651-7

Expedited Partner Therapy in the Management of STDs
H. Hunter Handsfield, Matthew Hogben, Julia A. Schillinger, Matthew R.
Golden,
Patricia Kissinger and P. Frederick Sparling
2010. ISBN: 978-1-60741-571-8

Periodontitis: Symptoms, Treatment and Prevention
Rosemarie E. Walchuck (Editor)
2010. ISBN: 978-1-61668-836-3
2010. ISBN: 978-1-61728-072-6 (E-book)

EMS Workforce for the 21st Century - A National Assessment
Javier C. Bailey (Editor)
2010. ISBN: 978-1-60741-998-3

Handbook of Disease Outbreaks: Prevention, Detection and Control
Albin Holmgren and Gerhard Borg (Editors)
2010. ISBN: 978-1-60876-224-8

Overweightness and Walking
Caleb I. Black (Editor)
2010. ISBN: 978-1-60741-298-4
2010. ISBN: 978-1-61668-516-4 (E-book)

Smoking Relapse: Causes, Prevention and Recovery
Johan Egger and Mikel Kalb (Editors)
2010. ISBN: 978-1-60876-580-5

Medicare Advantage: The Alternate Medicare Program
Charles V. Baylis (Editors)
2010. ISBN: 978-1-60876-031-2

Scientific and Ethical Approaches for Observational Exposure Studies
Alain E. Hughes (Editor)
2010. ISBN: 978-1-60876-034-3

Diabetes in Women
Eliza I. Swahn (Editor)
2010. ISBN: 978-1-61668-692-5
2010. ISBN: 978-1-61668-801-1 (E-book)

COPD Is/Is Not a Systemic Disease?
Claudio F. Donner (Editor)
2010. ISBN: 978-1-60876-051-0

Sepsis: Symptoms, Diagnosis and Treatment
Joseph R. Brown (Editor)
2010. ISBN: 978-1-60876-609-3
2010. ISBN: 978-1-61668-448-8 (E-book)

Breaking Down Barriers to Care:
Treating Tobacco Dependence in Vulnerable Populations
John E. Snyder and Megan J. Engelen
2010. ISBN: 978-1-60876-976-6

Controlling Disease Outbreaks: The Changing Role of Hospitals
Raoul E. Nap, Nico E.L. Meessen,
Maarten P.H.M. Andriessen and Tjip S. van der Werf
2010. ISBN: 978-1-61668-314-6
2010. ISBN: 978-1-61668-739-7 (E-book)

The H1N1 Influenza Pandemic of 2009
Charles R. Bartolotti (Editor)
2010. ISBN: 978-1-61668-357-3
2010. ISBN: 978-1-61668-392-4 (E-book)

Beyond the Words: Communication and Suggestion in Medical Practice
Katalin Varga (Editor)
2010. ISBN: 978-1-61668-590-4
2010. ISBN: 978-1-61728-084-9 (E-book)

Therapeutic Ultrasound: Mechanisms to Applications
Victor Frenkel (Editor)
2010. ISBN: 978-1-61668-599-7
2010. ISBN: 978-1-61728-076-4 (E-book)

Complementary and Alternative Medicine among Chinese Canadians
Marilyn A. Roth and Karen M. Kobayashi
2010. ISBN: 978-1-61728-014-6

PUBLIC HEALTH IN THE 21ST CENTURY

MRSA (METHICILLIN RESISTANT *STAPHYLOCOCCUS AUREUS*) INFECTIONS AND TREATMENT

MANAL M. BADDOUR

Professor of Medical Microbiology and Immunology
Faculty of Medicine, Alexandria University
Alexandria, Egypt

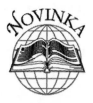

Nova Science Publishers, Inc.
New York

LIBRARY OF CONGRESS CATALOGING-IN-PUBLICATION DATA

MRSA (methicillin resistant Staphylococcus Aureus) infections and treatment /Author, Manal M. Baddour.
x, 128 p. ; 23 cm.
Includes bibliographical references (p. [83]-118) and index.
ISBN: 978-1-61668-038-1 (softcover)
1 .Staphylococcus aureus infections. 2.Methicillin resistance. I. Baddour, Manal M.
QR201.S68 B32 2010
(OCoLC)ocn505420624

2010283138

Published by Nova Science Publishers, Inc. † New York

PREFACE

Incidents of methicillin-resistant *Staphylococcus aureus* (MRSA) have been prominent in the news over the past few years, drawing attention to a type of infection that is resistant to certain antibiotics. *Staphylococcus aureus* has three features that make it distinct among most other clinically important bacteria. Not only do MRSA infections lead to higher lengths of stay and more cost than MSSA infections, but more importantly, MRSA infections lead to a higher mortality. It has been contended that the introduction of methicillin put an end to the tremendous amount of research and enthusiasm for the infection control measures which were effective and vigorous at the time when it was first introduced. The medical community experienced a false sense of security against these resistant pathogens. Once you could treat these previously antibiotic-resistant staphylococci, people stopped washing their hands and doing all the other things they now realize they should have been doing all along. MRSA is no longer confined to hospitals and hospital-attending people, it has now vigorously invaded recreational, rehabilitation, sporting and teaching facilities. Although the epidemiologic patterns of hospital acquired MRSA and community acquired MRSA may be dissolving, there remain clinical differences that, if unrecognized by the clinician, could cause delay in appropriate treatment and management.

What is MRSA, where did it come from? Did we bring it about by ourselves? Is it treatable? Is it truly deadly or are we overdoing it?

Chapter 1

INTRODUCTION AND TAXONOMY

Staphylococci are Gram-positive spherical bacteria that occur in microscopic clusters resembling bunches of grapes. They are aerobic or facultatively anaerobic, nutritionally undemanding and catalase-positive. Today, according to the current List of Bacterial Names with Standing in Nomenclature (Euzéby, 2004), the genus Staphylococcus comprises 36 species, eleven of which also contain subdivisions with named subspecies. The classification is still developing.

On the basis of comparative 16S rRNA sequence studies, the genus Staphylococcus belongs to the Gram-positive bacteria with a low DNA G+C content. They are closely related to bacilli and other Gram-positive bacteria with low DNA G+C content such as macrococci, enterococci, streptococci, lactobacilli and listeria. Combining Staphylococcus, Gemella, Macrococcus and Salinicoccus within the family Staphylococcaceae has been suggested (Garrity and Holt, 2001).

The Staphylococcus genus is ubiquitously distributed in nature, with some species inhabiting specific ecological niches. Staphylococci are found living naturally on the skin and mucous membranes of warm-blooded animals and humans (in fact, 25-30% of humans carry Staphylococci in their nares), but are also isolated from a wide range of foodstuffs such as meat, cheese and milk, and from environmental sources such as soil, sand, air and water (Kloos and Schleifer, 1986).

Most staphylococci species are coagulase-negative. Exceptions are *Staphylococcus aureus, Staphylococcus intermedius, Staphylococcus delphini, Staphylococcus schleiferi* subsp. *coagulans, Staphylococcus lutrae* and some strains of *Staphylococcus hyicus* (Kloos and Bannerman, 1995).

Staphylococcus aureus (*S. aureus*) was discovered in the 1880s. Since then, it has been shown to be a potential pathogenic Gram-positive bacterium, causing such infections as minor skin infections and post-operative wound infections. In the early 1940s, prior to the introduction of penicillin for the treatment of *S. aureus* infections, the mortality rate of individuals with an *S. aureus* infection was about 80% (Skinner and Keefer, 1941). In 1942, only two years after the introduction of penicillin for medical use, the first penicillin resistant *S. aureus* isolate was observed in a hospital. Later on, penicillin-resistant *S. aureus* strains were also observed in the community. Since 1960, around 80% of all *S. aureus* strains are resistant to penicillin. In 1961, 2 years after the introduction of methicillin, a penicillinase-resistant penicillin, *S. aureus* developed methicillin-resistance due to the acquisition of the *mec A* gene (Jevons, 1961).

The prevalence of methicillin resistant *S. aureus* (MRSA) isolates slowly increased over the next three decades, with the majority of isolates being hospital-associated. This started to change in 1982 with an outbreak of MRSA among intravenous drug users (Saravolatx *et al.,* 1982). During the last 45 years, various hospital-associated methicillin resistant *S. aureus* (HA-MRSA) clones disseminated worldwide. The predominant pattern of MRSA in the 1980s and 1990s remained a hospital-acquired disease with traditional risk factors (Brumfit & Hamilton-Miller, 1989; Lowy, 1998). MRSA has emerged epidemiologically in a similar manner to penicillin resistance in the 1950s, occurring first in health care-associated settings then in the community.

Epidemiological studies suggest that hospitals are the primary MRSA reservoir and that hospital contact account for most MRSA infections (Salgado *et al.,* 2003). Three major reservoirs of HA-MRSA within the hospital are patients, health care workers, and inanimate environment. Patients and health care workers may become colonized with MRSA and therefore serve as sources of transmission. The major cause of spread of infection is infection control lapses by health care professionals. Patients with nasal colonization at hospital admission appear to be at increased risk for subsequent infection with the same isolate. Between 10% and 30% of hospitalized patients who acquire MRSA will develop an HA-MRSA infection (Davis *et al.,* 2004; Huang & Platt, 2003).

Not only do MRSA infections lead to higher lengths of stay and more cost then MSSA infections, but more importantly, MRSA infections lead to a higher mortality (Crowcroft & Catchpole, 2002; McHugh & Riley, 2004). A 2003 meta-analysis that included 31 studies showed a significant increase in mortality with MRSA bacteremia compared with MSSA bacteremia (Cosgrove *et al.,* 2003). Mortality among patients with *S. aureus* surgical site infections was increasingly higher when compared with uninfected patients (mortality 2.1%), MSSA-infected patients (mortality 6.7%), and MRSA-infected patients (mortality 20.7%) ($P < 0.001$) (Engeman *et al.* ,2003). A delay in initiation of therapy is associated with a further increase in mortality, making it more important for clinicians to have a heightened awareness for MRSA infection and to be prepared to treat it (Lodise & McKinnon, 2005).

MRSA is largely clonal, with mutation being its main developmental mechanism. Scientists in the field go a long way to de-demonising MRSA as a so-called 'superbug' and reinforce the fact that MRSA are merely pathogenic bacteria which have responded to the intensive antibiotic selective pressure via a classical Darwinian survival process.

Chapter 2

THE CASE FOR MRSA

Staphylococcus aureus (*S. aureus*) is a major cause of nosocomial infection and is responsible for significant morbidity, mortality and an extended hospital stay (Steinberg *et al.,* 1996; Kluytmans *et al.,* 1997; Fowler & Sexton, 2001). Methicillin-resistant *Staphylococcus aureus* (MRSA) is associated with increased mortality, morbidity and length of stay as compared to methicillin-sensitive *Staphylococcus aureus* (MSSA). In 1974, the Centers for Disease Control and Prevention (CDC) estimated that 2 percent of the staph infections occurring in medical facilities were cases of MRSA; in 2004, the estimate had risen almost to 63 percent. In 2005, MRSA was found to be responsible for 94,360 infections and 18,650 deaths in the United States alone thereby killing more people than AIDs. It appears that nearly five percent of patients in United States hospitals may have acquired a particular antibiotic resistant staph infection, according to a nationwide survey conducted by the Association for Professionals in Infection Control and Epidemiology (APIC). Researchers surveyed a total of 1,200 hospitals and other health care facilities from all 50 states, and found 8,000 patients infected or colonized with MRSA, or 46 out of every 1,000. This suggests that up to 1.2 million hospital patients across the country may be infected every year. Knowledge about the nature and number of MRSA clones that are disseminating is required to implement any strategies to control the transmission of MRSA, either within hospitals, nursing homes, or the community. For this reason, rapid identification of MRSA strains is an important issue.

It has traditionally been accepted that hospital acquired MRSA (HA-MRSA) strains are usually associated with infections involving catheter lines (blood stream), urinary tract, surgical wound infections, ulcers, ventilator associated pneumonia, and biomedical prostheses (Graffunder & Venezia, 2002). This is in contrast to community acquired MRSA (CA-MRSA) strains, which are overwhelmingly associated with skin and soft tissue infections.

For clinicians, early recognition of MRSA infections is critical to assure prompt initiation of appropriate antibiotic therapy. Failure to recognize risk factors for MRSA can lead to delay in appropriate treatment, which can have devastating consequences.

S. aureus infection studies suggest that MRSA infection usually follows prior carriage rather than occurring from direct transmission during invasive procedures by staff or from the ICU environment (von Eiff *et al.*, 2001; Chang *et al.*, 1998). These data support the view that prevention of colonization of ICU patients with MRSA could reduce the frequency of MRSA infections (Keshtgar *et al.*, 2008). Colonized patients are those who are found to be carrying the bacteria in or on their bodies, but who have not shown any symptoms of disease. Colonization with MRSA may be an even greater risk factor for *S. aureus* skin and soft tissue infections than with MSSA colonization (Ellis *et al.*, 2004). Carriage of CA-MRSA has been implicated as a risk factor in several of the diverse settings in which outbreaks have occurred. However, MRSA nasal colonization is not invariably present in patients with active MRSA infections. The role of antecedent nasal colonization as a prelude to clinical infection is less clear in community acquired infections than in health care-associated infections (Moellering, 2006; Kazakova *et al.*, 2005; Ellis *et al.*, 2004; Adcock *et al.*, 1998). There are data to suggest that colonization in non-nasal sites is more common in CA-MRSA than MSSA or HA-MRSA (Yang *et al.*, 2007). This is in contrast to the 1% of non-nasal carriage seen with MSSA or HA-MRSA and suggests that skin-to-skin transmission may play a larger role in CA-MRSA infections (Miller & Diep, 2008). This may be due in part to the ability of these strains to colonize other unsampled tissue sites (e.g., vagina, rectum, or skin) (Cook *et al.*, 2007) and such sites may play a more important role in community-based infections than in health care-associated infections.

Reservoirs for MRSA include three major foci: patients and their families and pets, inanimate environment, and caregivers (Maki, 1978). The role of healthcare workers in MRSA control is undeniable for many reasons, and the potential for healthcare workers to directly or indirectly propagate MRSA is real although situationally variable (Cimolai, 2008). The main transmission of *S. aureus* occurs through direct hand contact from patient to personnel to patient or from patient to patient (Solberg, 2000); however, the relative importance of different modes of *S. aureus* transmission are continuously reviewed. In terms of indirect spreading from contaminated inanimate objects, a high resistance of MRSA on dry surfaces has been shown (Huang *et al.*, 2006; Dietze *et al.*, 2001; Wagenvoort *et al.*, 2000; Oie and Kamiya, 1996). Additionally, airborne transmission has been discussed (Mortimer *et al.*, 1996; Shiomori *et al.*, 2002). An increased awareness and use of infection control practices has had some impact on the prevalence of nosocomial infections. Isolation and decolonization of carriers and frequent hand-washing by healthcare workers as well as the use of dedicated care bundles have proven to be successful in reducing MRSA bacteraemia rates, but MRSA colonization rates remain high in many units and additional strategies for reducing MRSA rates are required (O'Hanlon & Enright, 2009).

Chapter 3

PREVALENCE AND EPIDEMIOLOGY

Staphylococcus aureus has three features that make it distinct among most other clinically important bacteria. It can express a variety of virulence factors, it has the ability to develop and expand resistance to a broad spectrum of antimicrobial drug classes, and it is prominent in both hospital and community settings (Flynn & Cohen, 2008; Styers *et al.,* 2006).

The epidemiology of *S. aureus* and in particular of MRSA is changing rapidly. Healthcare-associated MRSA is now endemic throughout the world and is a major cause of morbidity and mortality and excess healthcare costs (Gould, 2006; Grundmann *et al.,* 2006). MRSA is carried, or "colonized," by about 1% of the population, although most of them are not infected. The prevalence of MRSA increased dramatically in many countries during the 1990s. In the UK, MRSA bacteraemia (as a percentage of *S. aureus* bacteraemia) rose from <2% in 1990 to 43% in 2001 (Johnson *et al.,* 2005; Health Protection Agency, 2005) and this trend was mirrored in other countries including the USA and Japan.

Community-acquired MRSA infections have risen dramatically in prevalence in some countries, most notably in the USA (Moran *et al.,* 2006). These infections are caused by MRSA clones that are genetically distinct from those that are endemic in hospitals and they tend to infect younger individuals with few of the risk factors associated with nosocomial MRSA bacteraemia (Vidal *et al.,* 2009). In 2008, MRSA has evolved to be commonplace in the community and hospital setting. Currently, the majority of community-associated strains reported worldwide are methicillin-resistant (Moran *et al.,* 2006). Although the epidemiologic lines are beginning to blur, MRSA infections are still categorized as either health care- or community-associated infections (Byers *et al.*, 2008).

The National Nosocomial Infections Surveillance System reported that the proportion of HA-MRSA infections in U.S. hospital intensive care units (ICUs) increased from 35.9% in 1992 to 64.4% in 2003, an overall increase of 3.1% annually. It is predicted that, if this trend continues, the rate will reach 80% by 2010 (Klevenns *et al.*, 2006).

However, the MRSA prevalence between the countries in Europe is variable. The MRSA prevalence in the northern countries is approximately 1%, whereas the MRSA prevalence in the southern countries is as high as 45% (Tiemersma *et al.*, 2004).

During 2008, some countries have witnessed the first ever significant fall in the rate of healthcare-acquired MRSA bacteraemia, despite concern that this was essentially unachievable (Duckworth, 2005). It causes one-fifth of nosocomial infections in the UK and up to one in six patients in UK intensive care unit (ICU) wards are colonized or infected with MRSA. These strains are usually EMRSA-15 and -16, the most prevalent epidemic MRSA strains in the UK (Hails *et al.*, 2003; Moore & Lindsay, 2002; Johnson *et al.*, 2001; National Audit Office, 2000).

The highest MRSA rates in Europe (ca. 50%) are exceeded in many countries around the world, including the USA, Taiwan, Hong Kong, Singapore and Japan. Much of South America and the Middle East also have a major problem.

The Mediterranean region has been identified as an area of hyper-endemicity for multi-resistant hospital pathogens (Gur & Unal, 2001). This is clearly the case for MRSA within the European continent, where data from the European Antimicrobial Resistance Surveillance System (EARSS) indicate that almost all of the high prevalence countries border the Mediterranean sea (Tiemersa *et al.*, 2004). Other Mediterranean countries also suffer from this increased prevalence.

A possible measurable factor behind the documented prevalence of MRSA in the southeastern Mediterranean region could be infrastructural deficits related to inadequate bed availability to cope with peak demands, resulting in overcrowding. In addition, inadequate isolation facilities could be a further driver to compound these problems. Furthermore studies show that the mere presence of infection control teams, suitable hand hygiene facilities, as well as antibiotic stewardship initiatives does not necessarily guarantee adequate control of multiresistant infections such as MRSA. This could well be the result of the interplay of other confounding factors as well as possible underlying socio-cultural circumstances (Borg *et al.*, 2008).

Chapter 4

HOSPITAL ACQUIRED AND
COMMUNITY ACQUIRED

Community acquired MRSA's (CA-MRSA) time in the public eye has been short compared to the 62 years since bacteriologist Mary Barber confirmed the first instances of penicillin-resistant *S. aureus* at London's Hammersmith Hospital (Barber, 1947), or the 48 years since Barber's colleague Patricia Jevons reported the first signs of staphylococcal resistance to the synthetic penicillin replacement methicillin and related beta lactam antibiotics (Jevons, 1961). At the moment, the distinction between CA-MRSA and HA-MRSA is beginning to fade (Lowy, 1998, 2003).

The definitions of HA-MRSA and CA-MRSA are changing, and many different definitions can be found in the literature. In a meta-analysis of 32 studies, at least 8 definitions for CA-MRSA have been reported (Salgado *et al.*, 2003). They are defined by either the epidemiological setting where the infection occurs or by the molecular background of the infecting strains. There appears to be a merging of strains, which makes the definition and distinction even more challenging (Kourbatova *et al.*, 2005).

Two primary factors currently used in the categorization of MRSA infections are *time of infection isolation* and the presence or absence of *MRSA-related risk factors* (Generally, MRSA strains isolated after 48 to 72 hours of admission to a health care facility, or those present at the time of admission in recently discharged patients or residents of long-term care facilities, are interchangeably referred to as *nosocomial*, *hospital acquired*, *hospital-associated*, or *health care–associated* MRSA (HA-MRSA).

Terms used to describe cases of infection not involving a traditional health care setting (CA-MRSA) include *community-acquired, community-associated,* and *community-onset*. Of these, *community-onset* is generally used to refer to infections that begin outside of the health care setting (regardless of the presence of risk factors for MRSA), while infections occurring in a community setting in the absence of risk factors for MRSA are considered by some to represent cases of "true" CA-MRSA (Padmanabhan & Fraser, 2005).

Current criteria set forth by the Centers for Disease Control and Prevention (CDC, 2007) for distinguishing CA-MRSA from HA-MRSA state that patients with CA-MRSA infection tend to have all of the following characteristics:

- Diagnosis of MRSA made in the outpatient setting or on the basis of a positive culture for MRSA within 48 hours after hospital admission
- No medical history of MRSA infection or colonization
- No history in the preceding year of hospitalization, dialysis, surgery, or admission to a nursing home, skilled nursing facility, or hospice
- No permanent indwelling catheters or medical devices that pass through the skin into the body.

However, CA-MRSA can also be defined based on genetic markers, such as the presence of *SCCmec* type IV, V or VII and the presence of PVL. In addition, it has been reported that CA-MRSA is associated with several specific *S. aureus* lineages (Tristan *et al.,* 2007). A recent study showed that defining CA-MRSA by the absence of risk factors for healthcare exposure greatly underestimates the burden of epidemic CA-MRSA disease (David *et al.,* 2008).

Community-acquired strains of MRSA are distinct from HA-MRSA strains from genotypic, phenotypic, and epidemiologic perspectives (Hisata *et al.,* 2005; Vandenesch *et al.,* 2003; Daum *et al.,* 2002; Daum, 1998). At a genetic level, CA-MRSA is more similar to methicillin-susceptible *S aureus* (MSSA) than to traditional MRSA, and its emergence appears to be due to the acquisition, by an MSSA strain, of the staphylococcal cassette chromosome (SCC) carrying *mecA*, the gene encoding the methicillin-resistant penicillin binding protein (Robinson *et al.,* 2005). The majority of the studies have described that PVL, together with *SCCmec* type IV or V and a specific genetic background, is a genetic marker for CA-MRSA (Tristan *et al.,* 2007). It is also found to infect much younger people. In a study from Minnesota, USA, published in The Journal of the American Medical Association, the average

age of people with MRSA in a hospital or healthcare facility was 68. But the average age of a person with CA-MRSA was only 23.

In a 2003 meta-analysis of 27 retrospective and 5 prospective studies, CA-MRSA was found to account for 30.2% and 37.3%, respectively, of MRSA isolates from hospitalized patients (Salgado *et al.,* 2003). While a large majority (85%) of these patients had one or more health care-associated risk factors for MRSA (Salgado *et al.,* 2003), the remainder represent cases of "true" CA-MRSA.

In a more recent study that included 319 patients with CA-MRSA infection who presented to one of several rural hospitals in Idaho or Utah, USA, 75% of these patients did not have any identified risk factor for MRSA (Stevenson *et al.,* 2005). Another study from a single medical center in Atlanta evaluated 384 persons with microbiologically confirmed community-onset *S. aureus* skin infections, of which 72% were due to MRSA (King *et al.,* 2006). Among all *S. aureus* isolates, 63% were considered to be community-acquired and 99% were the USA 300 clone. This rate of CA-MRSA represents a much higher percentage than reported in the meta-analysis and suggests that the actual incidence of CA-MRSA is increasing.

Thus the hospital acquired disease pattern associated with MRSA started to change in 1982 with an outbreak of community acquired-MRSA (CA-MRSA) among intravenous drug users. This trend continued with a shift toward more community-acquired infections and was highlighted in the 2006 EMERGEncy ID Net Study, which demonstrated that MRSA was the most common identifiable cause of skin and soft tissue infections among patients who presented to emergency departments in 11 U.S. cities. The overall prevalence of MRSA in this population was 59% (Moran *et al.,* 2006). Community acquired MRSA (CA-MRSA) has rapidly emerged in the community becoming an increasingly common etiologic agent in skin and soft tissue infections and has recently become the most common etiologic agent of these infections in many centers (Moran *et al.,* 2006). One study of children in south Texas found that cases of CA-MRSA had a 14-fold increase between 1999 and 2001. This increase in prevalence of CA-MRSA infections is rising both in terms of absolute numbers of cases admitted to hospitals and as a proportion of all cases of MRSA (Fridkin *et al.,* 2005; Eady & Cove, 2003).

Following the four paediatric deaths in Dakota and Minnesota, the emergence of MRSA in the community setting has become a major focal point of epidemiological research (King *et al.,* 2006; Kluytmens *et al.,* 2006; Rossney *et al.,* 2005; Vandenesch *et al.,* 2003; Okuma *et al.,* 2002; Anon, 1999; Lina *et al.,* 1999). MRSA clones of true community origin arise from the horizontal transfer of *mecA* into circulating methicillin-susceptible *S. aureus* strains and are typically characterized by the presence of *SCCmec* IV, susceptibility to non-β-lactams and the gene locus for Panton Valentine leukocidin (PVL) (Tenover *et al.*, 2006; Baba *et al.*, 2002; Lina *et al.*, 1999).

During the last decade, CA-MRSA has emerged worldwide, not only in the community, causing serious infections in people of all ages and backgrounds (Fridkin *et al.*, 2005), but also in healthcare facilities. In general, CA-MRSA is more virulent compared to HA-MRSA due the presence of various virulence factors (Etienne, 2005; Chambers, 2001). The emergence of virulent strains of MRSA in patients in the community who have none of the traditional risk factors for MRSA is extremely worrisome (Fridkin *et al.*, 2005).

The characteristics of HA-MRSA and CA-MRSA differ microbiologically and clinically. These differences are at a molecular level, the presence of specific virulence factors, exotoxin production, and antimicrobial susceptibilies (Diedren & Kluytmans, 2006). Strains of CA-MRSA are more frequently susceptible to a variety of non-beta-lactam antibiotics. CA-MRSA genotypically differs from HA-MRSA in that it carries *SCCmec* types IV or V and is associated with the genes encoding Panton-Valentine leukocidin (PVL) toxin (Deurenberg *et al.*, 2007). Although a small percentage contain *SCCmec* type V, these strains predominantly carry *SCCmec* type IV, which is smaller in size than the gene cassette found in most strains of HA-MRSA (types I, II, and III). This observed difference in SCC size may allow for more efficient transfer of resistance among different bacteria, a factor that may be relevant in the alarmingly rapid emergence of CA-MRSA.

The emergence of CA-MRSA and the growing presence of a community reservoir for methicillin-resistant strains threatens future control of antimicrobial resistance in the health care setting. Since CA-MRSA may now significantly contribute to nosocomial dissemination of MRSA within hospitals, the distinction between CA-MRSA and HA-MRSA within the hospital setting has become blurred. The migration of resistant strains from the community reservoir into hospitals is a potentially troubling development, and gradual increases in this community reservoir can be expected to lead to failure of traditional control measures. Recognition and isolation of symptomatic individuals, along with contact-tracing and quarantining, are two basic measures of control (Fraser *et al.*, 2004) that cannot be used effectively in a community setting. Isolation of infected individuals and carriers is much less manageable in a community setting compared with the relatively closed and controlled environment of the hospital. For this reason, the presence of a community reservoir from which resistant strains can recurrently be transmitted into the health care setting is a significant and growing challenge for the control of MRSA.

Its increase in the community is of additional concern because the CA-MRSA strains appear to be highly virulent, and colonization with CA-MRSA is often undetected in hospitalized patients, which can facilitate spread in the hospital and its potential for becoming resistant to multiple antibiotics.

CA-MRSA could likely have its origins in the health care setting. One source of MRSA in the community is attributed to escaped nosocomial isolates (particularly among people with traditional MRSA risk factors) in addition to the novel community isolates of MRSA. Nosocomial MRSA spreads within the community setting from patients at risk of MRSA carriage to individuals without recent recorded hospital contact. Patients discharged from the hospital often continue to be colonized with MRSA and may become reinfected or may transfer such strains to community contacts. MRSA-colonized patients can persist asymptomatically in 76% of people for up to 12 months. Thus, patients discharged from a hospital can function as reservoirs of MRSA in both the community and the health care-associated setting. Individuals with CA-MRSA then serve as an important reservoir for transmission and dissemination back into the hospital (Eady & Cove, 2003; Seybold *et al.,* 2006). In proof of such a perspective, phenotypical and genotypical analysis demonstrated that MRSA isolates retrieved from the West Midlands community in the UK were not characteristic of CA-MRSA. The majority of the isolates were related to hospital epidemic strains, demonstrating the probable transmission of MRSA from the hospital setting into the surrounding community. The predominance of MRSA isolates harbouring *SCCmec* IV among these demonstrates the transmissible success of *SCCmec* IV outside the hospital setting (Rollason *et al.,* 2008)

One CA-MRSA clone, designated USA300 by the CDC, was first isolated in the San Francisco area in 2000 (McDougal *et al.,* 2003). Despite multiple other strains of CA-MRSA circulating (USA400, USA1000, USA1100), USA300 predominates in outbreaks of skin and soft tissue infection (SSTI) (Kline *et al.,* 2006). Currently, it is unclear why one clone predominates, but most likely USA300 is uniquely adapted for ease of transmission in crowded settings.

It is likely that enzymes such as Toxic Shock Syndrome toxin 1, α-hemolysin, enterotoxins Q and K, staphylokinase, and other proteases are the more significant virulence factors in USA300 rather than PVL historically thought to be responsible for virulence. These toxins are also attributed to the necrotic appearance of CA-MRSA SSTI, which is commonly misdiagnosed as a brown recluse spider bite.

Characteristics of HA-MRSA and CA-MRSA are further differentiated by antimicrobial resistance patterns. Strains of CA-MRSA are more frequently susceptible to a variety of non-beta-lactam antibiotics. Multidrug resistance (MDR) MRSA isolates are a significant concern for HA-MRSA. HA-MRSA is associated with *SCCmec* types II and III and, thus, is significantly more likely to be resistant to >3 antibiotics (Charlebois *et al.*, 2002). Resistance to macrolides, clindamycin, and fluoroquinolones are common along with variable resistance to tetracycline and trimethoprim-sulfamethoxazole. HA-MRSA is usually susceptible to vancomycin and rifampin. Unlike HA-MRSA isolates, many CA-MRSA isolates to date have been resistant only to beta lactams (the antimicrobial class that includes penicillin and cephalosporins) and macrolides/azalides (eg, erythromycin, clarithromycin, azithromycin). However, resistance to other classes of antimicrobial agents, such as fluoroquinolones and tetracycline, occurs and may be increasing in prevalence (Baddour *et al.*, 2006). Most CA-MRSA isolates have been susceptible to trimethorpim-sulfamethoxazole, gentamicin, tetracycline, and clindamycin. Clones resistant to erythromycin can confer inducible resistance to clindamycin and have been reported in USA300 CA-MRSA isolates (Bradley, 2005). The generation of MDR CA-MRSA isolates will make it increasingly difficult for clinicians to choose the appropriate empiric antimicrobial therapy based on epidemiologic information. Although the epidemiologic patterns of HA-MRSA and CA-MRSA may be dissolving, there remain clinical differences that, if unrecognized by the clinician, could cause delay in appropriate treatment and management (Chavez *et al.*, 2008).

Chapter 5

DIFFERING SPECTRUMS OF DISEASE

It is important that clinicians be aware of the spectrum of disease caused by CA-MRSA, which differs from that of HA-MRSA in distribution and pattern of infection. Patients infected with CA-MRSA tend to be significantly younger than those infected with traditional strains of MRSA. Unlike traditional MRSA strains, which often are isolated from the bloodstream and the respiratory and urinary tracts, CA-MRSA strains are typically found on skin and in soft tissue and occur in settings that involve crowding, contact, and compromised hygiene (Salgado *et al.,* 2003). Interestingly, because skin infections due to CA-MRSA often have a necrotic center, many have been mistaken for spider bites.

A SSTI develops as a result of a combination of factors: the virulence of the organism, the tropism of the organism to the skin, and the presence of several host risk factors. The Centers for Disease Control and Prevention (CDC) defines CA-MRSA SSTI as a skin or soft tissue lesion occurring in a patient with symptoms such as pain, warmth, or pus, from which MRSA is cultured (CDC, 2001). The most commonly seen CA-MRSA SSTIs are cellulitis, folliculitis, and abscess. However, recent reports have implicated CA-MRSA as causing more invasive SSTI, such as necrotizing fasciitis and pyomyositis (Miller *et al.,* 2007; Fridkin *et al.,* 2005).

Outbreaks have been reported in specific geographic locations (Ma *et al.,* 2005; Peleg *et al.,* 2005; Ribeiro *et al.,* 2005; Schulz *et al.,* 2005; Iyer & Jones, 2004; Salgado *et al.,* 2003) and in several well defined and characteristically "closed" populations, including Alaskan natives, American Indians, children, participants in team sports, military personnel, and correctional facility inmates (Buescher, 2005; Cohen, 2005; Lu & Holton, 2005; Purcell & Fergie,

2005; Rihn *et al.*, 2005; Weber, 2005; Ellis *et al.*, 2004). CA-MRSA is now the predominant cause of community-associated skin infections (Moran *et al.*, 2006).

Although CAMRSA is primarily involved in skin and soft tissue infections, it has also been implicated in sepsis and necrotizing pneumonia (Francis *et al.*, 2005; Mongkolrattabithai *et al.*, 2003). Pneumonia associated with PVL producing MRSA is more frequently associated with sepsis, high fever, leukopenia, hemoptysis, pleural effusions, and death compared with PVL-negative MRSA strains (Boyle-Vavra & Daum, 2007). Recent in vitro work revealed that PVL toxin-producing MRSA binds preferentially to damaged respiratory epithelium, which correlates clinically with data showing that PVL associated pneumonias are associated with prior influenza-like illnesses (Gillet *et al.*, 2002).

Certain clones of MRSA may cause more severe invasive disease. The MRSA clone USA300 is responsible for the dramatic increase in MRSA disease in the United States and is considered the prototypical CA-MRSA strain. Rapid dissemination of this single clone is responsible for this epidemic (Liu *et al.*, 2008; Diep *et al.*, 2006a). Its unique molecular characteristics may also play a key role in pathogenesis. Not only does it possess PVL toxin, but it also has genomic adaptations (*SCCmec* type IV) that can enhance fitness by co-selecting for multidrug resistance and enhance growth and survival on the human skin (Diep *et al.*, 2008, 2006b).

Chapter 6

PANTON-VALENTINE LEUKOCIDIN

Since the 1990s, virulent CA-MRSA clones, characterized by the presence of the Panton-Valentine leukocidin (PVL), spread worldwide, first in the community, but later on also in healthcare facilities.

The PVL, having cytolitic activity against human and rabbit monocytes and polymorph nuclear cells, was first reported by Panton and Valentine in 1932 (Panton and Valentine, 1932). PVL is a staphylococcal membrane toxin that targets and kills leukocytes (Kline *et al.,* 2006). Historically, PVL was thought to be the primary virulence factor of CA-MRSA resulting in skin and soft tissue infections (SSTI) (Yamasaki *et al.,* 2005). However, recently it has been proposed that PVL serves as more of a marker of CA-MRSA virulence, and that other toxins played more of a role in the development of SSTI (Voyich *et al.,* 2006).

A total of 40–90% of MRSA strains carrying *SCCmec* type IV express PVL (Kourbatova *et al.,* 2005). This *S. aureus* -specific exotoxin has been associated with skin and soft tissue infections and severe necrotizing pneumonia (Vandenesch *et al.,* 2003). The toxin consists of two polypeptides, S- (slow-eluted) and F- (fast-eluted) components, based on their elution profiles through cation-exchange chromatography (Kaneko and Kamio, 2004; Noda and Kato, 1988; Woodin, 1960). PVL toxin is likely to be involved in severe symptoms such as necrotic pneumonia and furunculosis.

It is postulated that PVL contributes to enhanced community fitness, perhaps from enhanced transmission for draining wounds. It also may enhance the ability to initiate infection in intact skin, directly cause or exacerbate lesions, or facilitate local spread. CA-MRSA strains are also associated with production of other toxins, such as staphylococcal enterotoxin Q and K, α-hemolysin which are capable of causing illness resembling toxic shock syndrome in animal models and may play a role in severe human infections (Labandeira *et al.*, 2007).

Recently, a new class of secreted, short staphylococcal peptides called phenol-soluble modulin peptides, were found to be associated with virulence of CA-MRSA skin infections. These peptides recruit, activate, and lyse neutrophils, the main host defense response against *S. aureus* (Wang *et al.*, 2007).

Chapter 7

MECHANISM OF β-LACTAM
RESISTANCE IN MRSA

S. aureus is a dynamic and adaptable bacteria that has a remarkable ability to acquire antibiotic resistance quickly. The cell wall of Gram-positive bacteria is composed of a single, extensively cross-linked peptidoglycan macromolecule, which confers strength and rigidity, maintaining the bacterial shape and protecting against osmotic forces. Structurally, peptidoglycan (murein) is composed of polysaccharide chains of alternating N-acetylglucosamine and N-acetylmuramic acid sugar residues, which are cross-linked by peptide bridges. Its synthesis involves three distinct phases. The first phase, which occurs in the cytoplasm, involves sequentially adding amino acids (L-alanine, D-glutamine, L-lysine, and a dimer of D-alanine) to a UDP-linked N-acetylmuramic acid molecule. In the second phase, this sugar pentapeptide is transferred from the UDP molecule to a lipid carrier (bactoprenol), which transports it across the cytoplasmic membrane, where a further N-acetylglucosamine residue is linked to the N-acetylmuramic acid and, in staphylococci, the ε-amino group of the lysine residue is substituted by pentaglycine.

During the third phase, which occurs at the external surface of the cytoplasmic membrane, the resulting disaccharide-pentapetide is linked onto an existing polysaccharide chain in a reaction termed transglycosylation. Cross-linking of the polysaccharide chains then follows, with attachment via their peptide substituents. This step is catalysed by multiple D-alanyl-D-alanine transpeptidases. They, along with other penicillin susceptible (but non-critical) enzymes, are referred to as penicillin-binding proteins (PBPs) and are the key targets of β-lactam action. β-lactams owe their ability to inhibit these enzymes to a conformational resemblance to D-alanyl-D-alanine; in consequence, they irreversibly inhibit the D-alanyl-D-alanine transpeptidases by covalent acylation of an active site serine. *S. aureus* has three essential PBPs with transpeptidase activity, PBP1, PBP2 and PBP3, and all remain, unaltered, in MRSA (Livermore, 206). Rather, the resistance of MRSA to β-lactams is mediated by a supplementary peptidoglycan transpeptidase PBP, PBP2' (also known as PBP2a, 78KDa), which continues to function when the normal PBPs have been inactivated by β-lactams (de Lancastre *et al.,* 1994). PBP2' does bind some available β-lactams, but only with extremely weak affinity. All strains of MRSA produce this unique PBP (PBP2a) that confers resistance ranging from a few cells (heterogeneous resistance) to a majority of cells in a population (homogeneous resistance) (Chambers, 1997; Mulligan *et al.,* 1993).

It is encoded by an acquired gene, *mecA*, 2.1 kb in length ,which is invariably located on a poorly mobile genetic element termed the staphylococcal cassette chromosome mec (*SCCmec*), and which is inserted into the *S. aureus* chromosome at a specific, consistent position (Katayama *et al.,* 2000). The origin of *SCCmec* is not known. Wu et al. suggested that *Staphylococcus sciuri* harbored the ancestor of PBP2a, since it was shown that a PBP was present in *S. sciuri* that had a 87.8% amino acid sequence identity compared to PBP2a. These *S. sciuri* strains were methicillin susceptible, but in the presence of methicillin these strains became resistant to methicillin due to the increased rate of transcription of the *mecA* homologue. It seems that *SCCmec* moved from coagulase-negative staphylococci to *S. aureus* by horizontal transfer (Deurenberg *et al.,* 2007).

The *mecA* gene is regulated by the repressor *MecI* and the transmembrane β-lactam-sensing signal-transducer *MecR1*, which are both divergently transcribed. *MecI* represses both the transcription of *mecA* and *mecR1–mecI* in the absence of a β-lactam antibiotic. However, in the presence of a β-lactam antibiotic, *MecR1* is autocatalytically cleaved, and the metalloprotease domain, which is located in the cytoplasmic part of *MecR1*, becomes active. This metalloprotease cleaves *MecI*, which, in turn, is bound to the *mecA* operator region, allowing the transcription of *mecA*, and the subsequent production of PBP2a to occur (Berger-Bachi and Rohrer, 2002).

There are seven major staphylococcal cassette chromosome variants, differing in size and regulatory genes (Robinson & Enright, 2004). Their restriction to a relatively few clonal complexes of MRSA strains may be because these are the only lineages that are permissive of *mecA* and its product

(Ktayama *et al.*, 2000), or may simply reflect the rarity of transfer. Nevertheless, some horizontal transfer does occur, as evidenced by the facts that the same *SCCmec* variants occur in different clonal complexes, and that some MRSA and MSSA strains are clonally identical. Moreover, the same *SCCmec* variants occur in both MRSA and coagulase-negative staphylococci (Enright *et al.*, 2002; Fitzgerald *et al.*, 2001).

At the moment, seven main types of *SCCmec* (type I to VII) are recognized, which vary in size, genetic composition, and antimicrobial resistance patterns. *SCCmec* types range in size from 20.9 to 66.9 kb. *SCCmec* type I (34.3 kb), IV (20.9–24.3 kb), V (28 kb), VI (20.9 Kb), and VII (35.9 kb) cause only β-lactam antibiotic resistance, while *SCCmec* type II (53.0 kb) and III (66.9 kb) cause resistance to multiple classes of antibiotics, due to the additional drug resistance genes integrated into *SCCmec*, i.e. integrated plasmids, e.g. pUB110, pI258 and pT181, and two transposons, e.g. Tn554 and CTn554. Integrated plasmid pUB110 harbors the *ant(4')* gene, encoding resistance to several aminoglycosides, e.g. kanamycin, tobramycin and bleomycin. Resistance to penicillins and heavy metals, such as mercury, is encoded by pI258, while tetracycline resistance is encoded by pT181. Transposon Tn554 harbors the ermA gene, coding for constitutive and inducible macrolide, lincosamide and streptogramin (MLS) resistance, while CTn554 encodes for resistance to cadmium (Ito *et al.*, 2001, 2003; Leclercq, 2002; Oliveira *et al.*, 2006; Takano *et al.*, 2008). In addition to the resistance genes carried on *SCCmec*, *S. aureus* can also harbor resistance genes on other sites of the genome, such as Tn554, as well as on plasmids (Lindsay & Holden, 2006). It has been shown recently that *SCCmec* type III is a composite element that consists of two SCC elements, i.e. *SCCmec* type III and SCCmercury, harboring ccrC, pI258 and Tn554 (Chongtrakool *et al.*, 2006).

There is a relatively large number of *SCCmec* type IV variants compared to variants of the other *SCCmec* types which could be due to the relative high frequency of horizontal transfer of *SCCmec* type IV, and the genetic plasticity of the MRSA lineages carrying this element (Jansen *et al.*, 2006).

Evidence indicates that *SCCmec* type IV strains may be more fit for survival than other strains (Maree *et al.*, 2007). The smaller size of *SCCmec* type IV types make them more efficient in transfer by phages to MSSA and, along with rapid growth rates, facilitates the spread of MRSA, which may displace other MRSA strains in hospitals (Pan *et al.*, 2005).

Some *S. aureus* strains have a more subtle and less common type of oxacillin resistance that is unrelated to the presence of the *mecA* gene. The resistance mechanism in these isolates is due to either overproduction of β-lactamase or the presence of altered PBP not related to 2a or 2'. These isolates usually have MICs at or just above susceptibility break zones. The isolates are sometimes referred to as borderline-resistant *S. aureus* (BORSA). They are often susceptible to other anti-staphylococcal agents.

Chapter 8

MRSA COLONIZATION

The distinction between colonization and infection is important:

Colonization = the presence of the bacteria, but no signs of illness or infection. Staph thrives in warm, moist places; common sites of colonization include the nostrils, umbilicus, axilla and groin.

Infection = clinical signs of illness or inflammation (e.g., localized pain/tenderness, redness, warmth, swelling, pus, fever). These are due to tissue damage caused by invasion by the bacteria.

The anterior nares are the primary reservoir for *S. aureus*, where replication occurs followed by subsequent dispersal to the skin (Kluytmans *et al.*, 1997). This is supported by studies that show that, if *S. aureus* nasal carriage is eliminated by the use of intranasal mupirocin, colonization often simultaneously resolves from other body sites (Kluytmans *et al.*, 1997; Reagan *et al.*, 1991).

A major principle in the pathogenesis of MRSA infections is that MRSA colonization precedes infection (Mulligan *et al.*, 1993; Miller & Diep, 2008). In proof of this concept of the importance of nasal colonization in the pathogenesis of infection is that, when colonization is eradicated, the risk of clinical infection is lowered (Reagan *et al.*, 1991), which has spurred attempts to eradicate *S. aureus* from the nose to prevent infection among high-risk groups.

However, data from outbreaks of community-acquired MRSA infections suggest that skin-skin and skin-fomite contact represent important and common alternative routes in the acquisition of the infecting MRSA strain and nasal colonization may play a less important role. So the stepwise logical progression of colonization to infection may not occur in community-associated CA-MRSA (Miller & Diep, 2008).

Data that supports non-nasal colonization in the pathogenesis of CA-MRSA infection include outbreak investigations of CA-MRSA infections in football teams, which revealed that the responsible clone of MRSA was not found in the nares of infected players (Kazakova *et al.*, 2005; Begier *et al.*, 2004).

Another investigation found that patients with acute CA-MRSA infection were more likely to have colonization of sites other than nares (axillae, inguinal, and rectum), in contrast to patients with acute CA methicillin-susceptible *S. aureus* (MSSA), HA-MRSA, or HA-MSSA, where non-nasal colonization was rare (Yang *et al.*, 2007). The unique characteristics of CA-MRSA may lead to a different pathogenesis of infection compared with HA-MRSA and MSSA. In outbreaks involving athletic teams, CA-MRSA infections were associated with exposures to various contaminated fomites, such as shared razors, towels, soap bars, and whirlpools. In addition, reported skin-skin contact, especially contact with broken skin, which occurs during games and practices, facilitated the spread of infection (Kazakova *et al.*, 2005; Begier *et al.*, 2004).

Control measures are essential to limit and prevent the spread of MRSA in outbreaks. These measures may include isolation of patients with MRSA, screening of contact patients and staff, and temporary removal of colonized staff from the medical setting (Mulligan *et al.*, 1993). Because the health care staff colonized with MRSA are an important source of MRSA spread, it has been advocated that attempts should be made to decolonize them (Duckworth *et al.*, 1998). Various topical and oral agents have been used to eradicate MRSA colonization, and variable clearance rates have been achieved. In general, the results have been unsatisfactory, and relapse and recolonization have been reported. Because of the consequences of excessive use of vancomycin, it is probably undesirable to use this antibiotic in all colonized patients. One might use oral vancomycin only in patients with digestive tract colonization. However, oral vancomycin is not tolerated by all patients.

It has been emphasized that eradication of MRSA carriage is justified in outbreak situations in health-care settings (Fraise, 1998; Mulligan *et al.*, 1993). Several eradication regimens have been used. Topical agents alone or in combination with oral antibiotics have been used for the elimination of both nasal and extranasal MRSA carriage (Harbarth *et al.*, 1999; Parras *et al.*, 1995; Valls *et al.*, 1994; Walsh *et al.*, 1003; Darouiche *et al.*, 1991; Arathoon *et al.*, 1990; Peterson *et al.*, 1990; Bitar *et al.*, 1987). Intranasal application of mupirocin seems to be the most effective topical agent for the eradication of MRSA nasal carriage (Duckworth *et al.*, 1998; Hill *et al.*, 1998; Kauffman *et al.*, 1993). Relapse and recolonization, however, are still frequently reported, and clearance rates have often been unsatisfactory (Mulligan *et al.*, 1993). It also seems that excessive use of mupirocin has lead to a dramatic drop in susceptibility of MRSA isolates to this antibiotic (Baddour *et al.*, 2006). Several hospitals in the Netherlands use oral vancomycin in combination with topical agents for the eradication of MRSA colonization. One study showed the efficacy of the combination of oral vancomycin, topical intranasal mupirocin, and a bath with povidone-iodine shampoo in eliminating MRSA colonization (Maraha *et al.*, 2002).

In one study, topical application of 5% vancomycin for 2 weeks was successfully used to eradicate MRSA nasal carriage in two nurses (Bitar *et al.*, 1987). In another study, vancomycin ointment failed to eradicate nasal carriage of methicillin sensitive staphylococci (Bryan *et al.*, 1981). In two case reports, decolonization of nasopharyngeal MRSA colonization was achieved using a vancomycin aerosol (Gradon *et al.*, 1992; Weathers *et al.*, 1990).

Chapter 9

CLINICAL RELEVANCE OF CA-MRSA

In the mid-1990s, providers in the San Francisco region noted MRSA, an organism historically associated with nosocomial infections, causing SSTI and coined the term community-associated MRSA (CA-MRSA) (Charlebois *et al.*, 2004). Since then, the epidemic of CA-MRSA has spread throughout the United States, currently accounting for more than one-half of all SSTI-related *S. aureus* isolates in the outpatient setting (Moran *et al.*, 2006). A recent longitudinal analysis from 1996 to 2004 of all *S. aureus* infections within a large urban setting showed a dramatic increase in numbers of cases of CA-MRSA from 50 per year to an astonishing 1100 per year (Kline *et al.*, 2006).

Although CA-MRSA's time in the public eye has been short compared to the penicillin-resistant *S. aureus* or to the first report relating to the first signs of staph's resistance to the synthetic penicillin replacement methicillin and related β-lactam antibiotics (Jevons, 1961), it continues to make headlines because of large outbreaks in daycare centers and among members of athletic teams. CA-MRSA infections in children commonly lead to hospitalization. Life-threatening infections, such as necrotizing pneumonitis and brain abscess, can occur. The organism has crossed into hospitals and is now a common cause of hospital-acquired sepsis. Multidrug-resistant strains of MRSA are emerging in Asia, with the resistance based on either a novel gene cassette or a transmissible plasmid. The routine use of antibiotics in livestock seems to be contributing to the emergence of resistant organisms, and some of these have already produced human infection. Fortunately, most cutaneous CA-MRSA infections present as abscesses or furunculosis, and these manifestations generally respond to drainage. The recurrence and attack rates of close contacts are high and relate to persistent colonization. Although CA-MRSA can have dramatic presentations of hemorrhagic necrotizing pneumonia and death, it most commonly occurs as a SSTI in a young, otherwise healthy individual (Garnier *et al.,* 2006).

These data illustrate that the largest burden of illness is identified and treated by primary care and emergency room physicians. It is thus imperative that these clinicians have a high index of suspicion for MRSA so they can promptly initiate the appropriate antibiotic therapy. Failure to act quickly can lead to increased morbidity and mortality for patients. As more virulent strains and increasing resistance occur due to the dynamic nature of this pathogen.

Chapter 10

GISA VISA VRSA

Until now, glycopeptides and especially vancomycin, have been considered as the treatment of choice for MRSA infections. Vancomycin has been used successfully to treat infections with drug-resistant isolates of *S. aureus* for more than three decades. The drug has its limitations. In 1990, Kaatz *et al.*, described the first case of infection with a MSSA isolate with intermediate susceptibility to teicoplanin (TISA). Seven years later, the first infection caused by an MRSA isolate with intermediate susceptibility to vancomycin was reported in Japan (Hiramatsu *et al.*, 1997). Since then, at least 20 cases of infection caused by MRSA with intermediate susceptibility to both vancomycin and teicoplanin (GISA) have been reported worldwide from Japan, the USA, South America and many European countries (Denis *et al.*, 2002; Walsh *et al.*, 2002; Hood *et al.*, 2000; Hiramatsu *et al.*, 1997). Vancomycin-resistant *S. aureus* (VRSA) was first identified in Detroit, Michigan in 2002, mediated by the *vanA* gene complex acquired from vancomycin-resistant enterococci (CDC, 2002). Since then, seven cases of infections caused by VRSA have also been confirmed in the USA (Sievert *et al.*, 2008), and there are other unconfirmed reports from India. Nine VISA and one confirmed VRSA were reported to EARSS in 2006. Although VISA strains have hitherto been thought to be rare, a recent study from Turkey, in which 46 of 256 (18%) MRSA isolates obtained (mainly from blood and pus) between 1998 and 2002 showed the VISA phenotype, suggests that their incidence may be on the rise (Sancak *et al.*, 2005).

In addition to GISA, strains that are borderline-susceptible to glycopeptides, but exhibit low-frequency resistance to glycopeptides <10^6 subpopulation; hetero-GISA) have been described more frequently in Europe,

Brazil and Asia (Liu & Chambers, 2003; Denis *et al.*, 2002; Walsh *et al.*, 2002; Hiramatsu *et al.*, 1997). Although their clinical relevance is still questioned, such strains appear to be associated with a poor treatment outcome (Howden *et al.*, 2004; Fridkin *et al.*, 2003) and could represent the first step towards the emergence of glycopeptide-resistant mutants following further glycopeptides exposure (Hiramatsu, 2001).

Although the mechanisms underlying vancomycin resistance are not yet fully understood, changes to the bacterial cell wall—the site of action of the glycopeptides—are believed to be key. Vancomycin exerts its antimicrobial effect by inhibiting the cell-wall synthesis of *S aureus*. In contrast to β-lactams, glycopeptides bind to D-alanyl-D-alanine residues of the murein monomer. Binding of glycopeptides to the D-alanyl-D-alanine residues in the completed peptidoglycan layers does not inhibit nascent peptidoglycan synthesis, though it may interfere with crossbridge formation mediated by PBPs. This may be the reason why teicoplanin is synergistic with β-lactam antibiotics. If glycopeptides bind to murein monomers in the cytoplasmic membrane, peptidoglycan synthesis is completely inhibited, and the cells cease to multiply. However, for the glycopeptide molecules to bind to such targets, they have to pass through about 20 peptidoglycan layers without being trapped by the first targets. Since there are many D-alanyl-D-alanine targets in the peptidoglycan layers, many glycopeptide molecules are trapped in the peptidoglycan layers. This compromises the therapeutic effectiveness of glycopeptides. Mechanism of vancomycin resistance is suggested to be production of increased amounts of peptidoglycan. More murein monomers and more layers (probably 30–40 layers) of peptidoglycan are considered to be present in the cell wall. As a result, more vancomycin molecules are trapped in the peptidoglycan layers before reaching the cytoplasmic membrane where peptidoglycan synthesis occurs. This cell wall thickening is a cardinal feature of all vancomycin resistant isolates (Hiramatsu, 2001). This vancomycin trapping is designated "affinity trapping". Moreover, a higher concentration of vancomycin would be required to saturate all the murein monomers. Additionally, the mesh structure of the outer layers of thickened peptidoglycan is destroyed by the trapped vancomycin molecules themselves. This prevents further penetration of vancomycin molecules into the inner part of cell-wall layers (otherwise known as the "clogging" phenomenon) (Cui *et al.*, 2000). It has been suggested that VRSA isolates possess altered peptidoglycan which confers markedly decreased affinity for vancomycin binding (Sakoulas & Moellering, 2008).

A similar resistance mechanism to teicoplanin, the other glycopeptide, is to be expected. However, there appears to be an extra resistance mechanism that might be over-expression of PBP2′ leading to increase in the rate of cross-linking of cell-wall peptidoglycan (Hiramatsu, 2001).

Recent evidence also supports the transfer of genetic material among bacteria as contributing to the development of VRSA. Based on the cases identified to date, risk factors for the development of VRSA may include older age, compromised blood flow to the lower limbs, and the presence of chronic ulcers.

In recent years, the threat of increasing vancomycin resistance in the global *S. aureus* population has led to the development of novel antibiotics for the potential treatment of infections caused by staphylococci.

Chapter 11

LABORATORY DIAGNOSIS AND TYPING OF MRSA

Clinicians are encouraged to collect specimens for culture and antimicrobial susceptibility testing from all patients with suspected MRSA infections, in particular skin abscesses with severe local cellulitis and/or systemic signs of infection or a history suggesting connection to outbreak or cluster of infections. MRSA should be considered in other syndromes compatible with *S. aureus* infections. This is useful in not only the management of the patient but also to determine the local prevalence of MRSA and antimicrobial susceptibility (Gorwitz *et al.*, 2008). At the present time, there is no information to suggest that molecular typing or identification of toxin genes should impact clinical care or management decisions. The Centers for Disease Control states that it is not necessary to routinely collect nasal cultures in all patients presenting with possible MRSA infections.

Conventional methods for the laboratory detection of MRSA include disk diffusion testing, recommended by the National Committee for Clinical Laboratory Standards; broth microdilution minimum inhibitory concentration testing; and oxacillin agar screen test (NCCLS, 1998).

The performance of these tests may be erratic because factors such as inoculum size, incubation temperature, duration of incubation, and variability in culture conditions may affect phenotypic expression of resistance. Most MRSA strains are heterogeneously resistant to methicillin, so only a small proportion of the *S. aureus* colonies that grow from a clinical specimen may show resistance in standard laboratory tests. Although all bacterial cells in a pure culture of MRSA have the basic genetic ability to express their resistance to β-lactam antibiotics, the cells may not behave in a homogenous manner, and frequently only 1 cell in 10^4 to 10^8 display readily detectable resistance in response to oxacillin.

Consequently, if too few cells appear resistant, an oxacillin-resistant strain may go undetected. This property makes detection of MRSA difficult. This phenomenon, called heteroresistance, makes it necessary for labs to use special methods to ensure detection of MRSA. In vitro testing conditions can be modified to enhance the expression of oxacillin resistance, including lower incubation temperatures (30-35°C), final test reading after a full 24 hours of incubation, and higher salt concentrations (supplementation agar with 2-4% sodium chloride).In our hands, we have found that combining 2 of these phenotypic methods greatly improves the test sensitivity and specificity especially in highly heterogeneous populations (Baddour *et al.*, 2007a).

All strains of MRSA have the *mecA* gene, whereas susceptible strains do not. Amplification of genetic determinants by polymerase chain reaction (PCR) assays have been used successfully to amplify and detect *mecA* gene sequences from clinical isolates and to detect MRSA directly from clinical specimens within a few hours (Hueletsky *et al.*, 2004). As they become more widely available, such rapid molecular assays will potentially influence the diagnosis and management of MRSA infections. Isolates identified as borderline-resistant do not grow on oxacillin screen plates.

PBP2' latex-agglutination test (Oxoid) can be used to detect MRSA and is reported to be highly sensitive and specific. However, one report testing problem MRSA isolates (giving discrepant results with different phenotypic testing methods) found the latex agglutination test to be less sensitive and less specific than expected (Baddour *et al.*, 2007a).

Recently, a rapid diagnostic test **IDI-MRSA** (Infectio Diagnostic, Inc., Sainte-Foy, Canada), which uses a real-time polymerase chain reaction (PCR) method to detect MRSA from clinical swabs, has been developed. This method gives a result within **2 hours**. The IDI-MRSA assay utilises real-time PCR for the amplification of an MRSA-specific DNA sequence and uses fluorogenic target-specific hybridization with a molecular probe for the detection of the amplified MRSA DNA. The sequences targeted in this assay are within the *SCCmec* cassette, which carries the *mecA* gene. Target-specific primers within the assay bind to these sequences and generate an MRSA-specific amplicon during the PCR, which can be detected by a molecular probe (Warren *et al.*, 2004). The test has a sensitivity of 92.5% and a specificity of 96.4% (according to the IDI-MRSA manufacturer test assay product insert).

However, whilst technically demanding and more expensive than traditional techniques for patient screening, it did not lead to reduction in transmission of MRSA, possibly due to lapses in infection control practices (Keshtgar *et al.*, 2008).

It must be noted that the results of testing for clindamycin susceptibility in CA-MRSA may be misleading. CA-MRSA strains are often susceptible to clindamycin, but the emergence of resistance during therapy has been reported, especially among erythromycin-resistant strains.Treatment failures have been documented when MRSA isolates were reported as susceptible to clindamycin but resistant to erythromycin (Siberry *et al.*, 2003). A double-disk diffusion test (D zone test) should be performed to identify inducible clindamycin resistance in erythromycin resistant, clindamycin-susceptible *S. aureus* isolates (CLSI, 2007).

The rapid identification of a problem pathogen is imperative to implement appropriate infection control strategies. Controlling the spread of this pathogen by screening patients, personnel and the environment remains a high priority in infection control programs. Tracing the source and transmission routes of MRSA relies on typing methods as tools for the genetic characterization of isolates (Maquelin *et al.*, 2007). Using phenotypic methods, such as antibiotic resistance to type *S. aureus* is disadvantageous because of poor discrimination. The introduction of genotyping techniques has improved the discrimination of *S. aureus*, the most widely used technique being pulsed-field gel electrophoresis (PFGE).

PULSED-FIELD GEL ELECTROPHORESIS (PFGE)

PFGE is one of the most discriminative typing methods for *S. aureus* and it is therefore considered the golden standard to investigate MRSA outbreaks in hospitals, as well as hospital-to-hospital transmission of MRSA. It is the reference method for molecular strain typing of MRSA. In PFGE for *S. aureus*, the extracted chromosomal DNA is digested with the restriction enzyme *SmaI*, and the resulting DNA fragments (15 to 20 bands) are separated by agarose gel electrophoresis in an electric field with an alternating voltage gradient. The resulting banding patterns are analyzed using a special software package, such as Bionumerics, Quantity one or Gel Compar II, using Dice comparison and unweighted pair group matching analysis (UPGMA) settings according to the criteria of Tenover et al. (1995). Although technically demanding, time consuming and expensive, PFGE is a tool which provides highly reproducible restriction profiles representing the entire bacterial genome and is far more discriminatory than RAPD for staphylococci (Maslow *et al.*, 1993; Raimundo *et al.*, 2002). Several attempts have been made to harmonize PFGE protocols and to establish a common nomenclature, but they were of limited success when assessed by cost of analyses, reproducibility (Baddour *et al.*, 2007b) and speed.

MULTILOCUS SEQUENCE TYPING (MLST)

MLST has been proven to be an excellent method to study the molecular evolution of *S. aureus*. This method is based on the sequence analysis of fragments of seven *S. aureus* housekeeping genes, i.e. *arcC, aroE, glpF, gmk, pta, tpi* and *yqiL*, each approximately 500-bp in length. A distinct allele is assigned to each of the different sequences of each housekeeping gene. The alleles of the seven genes define the *S. aureus* lineage, resulting in an allelic profile designated sequence type (ST). The nomenclature of MRSA is currently based on the ST and the type of *SCCmec* element. Disadvantages of MLST are generally that it is expensive, laborious and time consuming. MLST defines unambiguous strain types and results can easily be exchanged between different laboratories (Enright and Spratt, 1999). However, it is a relatively expensive method and therefore not an option for many clinical laboratories (Olive and Bean, 1999).

TYPING OF THE SPA LOCUS

This single-locus sequence typing technique for *S. aureus* has become increasingly popular during recent years. The method determines the sequence variation of the polymorphic region X of the *S. aureus* protein A (spa) locus (Frenay *et al.*, 1996). The diversity of the spa gene, consisting mainly of a number of repeats of 24 bp in length, is attributed to point mutations, as well as to deletions and duplications of the repeats (Shopsin *et al.*, 1999; Kahl *et al.*, 2005). Spa typing has a discriminative power between that of PFGE and MLST (Malachowa *et al.*, 2005), and, it has been shown that spa typing, in contrast to PFGE and MLST, can be used to study both the molecular evolution as well as hospital outbreaks of MRSA (Koreen *et al.*, 2004). Since spa typing involves sequencing of only a single locus, spa typing, compared to MLST, is less expensive, less laborious and less time consuming.

SCCMEC TYPING

The structure of *SCCmec* can be determined with a number of PCR-based methods that have been developed during the last few years. However, when investigating the structure of *SCCmec* in the same MRSA isolate, different results were sometimes obtained using these methods (Shore *et al.*, 2005; Kim *et al.*, 2007). A disadvantage of these developed methods is that they determine different structural properties of *SCCmec*. Therefore, the need exists for developing a single, universal assay for the determination of the structure of *SCCmec*.

REPETITIVE SEQUENCE-BASED PCR (REP-PCR)

Repetitive sequence-based PCR (rep-PCR) uses primers that target non-coding repetitive sequences interspersed in bacterial and fungal genomes (Koeuth *et al.*, 1995; Stern *et al.*, 1984; Versalovic *et al.*, 1991). When separated by electrophoresis, the amplified DNA fragments constitute a genomic fingerprint that can be employed for subspecies discrimination and strain delineation of bacteria and fungi (Versalovic and Lupski, 2002). The development of a commercially available, automated rep-PCR assay system, the DiversiLab System (bioMérieux, Boxtel, The Netherlands), offers advances in standardization and reproducibility over manual fingerprint generating systems (Healy *et al.*, 2005). The resulting DNA fingerprint patterns are viewed on a personal DiversiLab website as electropherograms. The software uses the Pearson correlation coefficient to analyze and calculate genetic similarity coefficients among all samples. The unweighted pair-group methods of averages (UPGMA) is employed to automatically compare the rep-PCR profiles and create corresponding dendrograms (Healy *et al.*, 2005). DiversiLab is rapid and non labor-intensive with the advantage of user-friendly web-based software. However, it lacks resolution to differentiate genetically and epidemiologically unique MRSA strains, needed for outbreak analysis.

RANDOMLY AMPLIFIED POLYMORPHIC DNA (RAPD)-PCR

Randomly amplified polymorphic DNA (RAPD)-PCR uses short primers with an arbitrary sequence to amplify genomic DNA. These primers randomly hybridize with chromosomal sequences that vary among different strains and that produce different amplification products. These products can be separated by gel electrophoresis to produce fingerprints or patterns characteristic of different epidemiological types (Casey *et al.*, 2007; Tambic *et al.*, 1999; Tang *et al.*, 1997). In comparison to other typing techniques, RAPD is overall a more rapid typing technique, although extracting DNA from staphylococcal isolates for RAPD can be time-consuming.

The method is relatively easy to perform and it is advisable to perform multiple tests with different primers (Cheeseman *et al.*, 2007). It has been claimed to confirm the clonal relationships as determined by PFGE and the Tenover criteria (Casey *et al.*, 2007). The fact that this technique can be used to type many other bacteria and yeasts makes it especially attractive for use in clinical laboratories. Moreover the discriminative power, reproducibility and rapidity of the method and its cost-effectiveness make it a candidate for use as a preventive diagnostic test (Herrera *et al.*, 2004; Hahn *et al.*, 2003; Tang *et al.*, 1997). Nevertheless, the ability of some RAPD methods to discriminate between staphylococcal strains has been debated (Saulinier *et al.*, 1993). Not only that, but acquisition or loss of individual resistance gene clusters or point mutations leading to adaptive resistance will go undetected by RAPD profiling, which only samples a small portion of the genome via PCR amplification to derive a genetic strain type and the reliance on a one-primer approach may not be sufficiently discriminatory.

Recently, an oligonucleotide array called "Staph.Array" has been developed, which targets the manganese-dependant superoxide dismute (*sodA*) gene (Giammarinaro *et al.*, 2005). It is the only tool described to date that distinguishes the 36 validated staphylococcal species in one shot and allows rapid, accurate identification of staphylococcal strains from clinical and food origins.

CA-MRSA has traditionally been distinguished from nosocomial MRSA by distinct epidemiologic and molecular differences noted in the organisms specifically USA300 pulsed-field gel electrophoresis (PFGE) strain type, presence of the PVL gene, and diminished antimicrobial resistance (Baba *et al.*, 2002). Over the last few years, new data on the evolving epidemiology of

S. aureus and CA-MRSA (Huang *et al.,* 2007, Mwangi *et al.,* 2007), as well as on the appearance and transmission of the organism in the health care setting (Bratu *et al.,* 2005; Saiman *et al.,* 2003), have blurred these distinctions.

Despite some success with MRSA rates in 2008, the original 'superbug' remains one step ahead of us. Its genomic plasticity (Dancer, 2008), ubiquitous existence, longevity and prominent human niche virtually guarantee long-term survival. No biological agent cannot be manipulated by the organism, despite the resilience of certain antibiotics, disinfectants and heavy metal ions (Crawford, 2008). Surveillance remains key for the spur required to search for alternative prevention and control measures.

Chapter 12

RISK FACTORS FOR HA-MRSA

MRSA acquisition has traditionally been linked to health care settings (eg, hospitals, long-term care facilities, dialysis centers) and specific patient populations eg, patients with prolonged hospital stay (14 days), previous antimicrobial use (especially cephalosporins or fluoroquinolones), presence in an ICU or burn unit, indwelling catheters, decubitus ulcers and postoperative surgical wounds, use of intravenous drugs, treatment with enteral feedings or dialysis, and the proximity to a patient colonized or infected with MRSA (Lodise, 2003; Graffunder & Venezia, 2002; Karchmer, 2000).

Nosocomial infection (i.e., hospital-onset) is defined by an MRSA-positive culture of a sample obtained >48 h after admission. Health care-associated infections have been defined previously (Chaves *et al.*, 2005; Buckingham *et al.*, 2004; Herold *et al.*, 1998), and include nosocomial infections or the presence of any of the following health care-associated risk factors within the year prior to a positive culture:

- Receipt of systemic antimicrobial treatment
- Residence in a long-term care facility (e.g. nursing home)
- Prior admission to an acute care facility, regardless of the duration of hospitalization (excluding clinic visits)
- Use of central intravenous catheters or long-term venous access devices
- Use of urinary catheters
- Use of other long-term percutaneous devices (i.e., thoracostomy tubes, nephrostomy tubes, biliary drains, percutaneous endoscopic gastrostomy tubes, traction pins, and external fixtures)

- Prior surgical procedures
- Undergoing any form of dialysis
- Close proximity to a patient in the hospital colonized with MRSA (Boyce, 1989)

In a study of MRSA bacteraemia applying the above mentioned criteria, it was found that wound infection was the most common source of MRSA bacteraemia in the study cohort, whereas the use of intravenous catheters, previous use of antibiotics and recent hospital admission were the most common predisposing factors. The mortality rate within 90 days was high (33%), similar to other published findings (Klein *et al.*, 2007). In addition to burn wounds, intubation was the primary focus of infection for burn patients with bacteraemia (Gang *et al.*, 2000).

Several researchers have studied hand hygiene compliance within the healthcare setting and judging by these studies, it appears that several factors have to do with hand hygiene compliance and can be summarized in the following: (Bell, 2006; Gordin *et al.*, 2005; Montville *et al.*, 2002; Boyce *et al.*, 2000).

Factors favouring hand hygiene compliance were:

- Convenient and accessible hand-hygiene facilities
- Preparations with good tolerability
- Perceived effectiveness of alcohol based hand rub vs standard hand washing
- High risk of transferring infectious agents
- Perceived benefit for patient
- Being female
- Educational background
- Being a nurse

Whereas factors hindering hand hygiene compliance were:

- Being a doctor
- Being male
- Working in high demand and stress environment
- Working on a weekday
- Wearing gloves or gowns
- Skin irritation

- Inaccessible supplies
- Too busy or lack of time
- Inconveniently located sinks
- Insufficient number of sinks
- Low risk of acquiring infection from patient
- Interference with patient-worker relationship
- Forgetfulness
- Ignorance of or disagreement with guidelines
- Perceived ineffectiveness of alcohol based hand rub vs standard hand washing

Following the introduction of (i) a reduction target, (ii) encouragement of hand hygiene by healthcare workers, and (iii) improving infection prevention surrounding insertion and care of indwelling lines and catheters, the MRSA bacteraemia episode rate per 1000 patient-bed-days has decreased in most National Health Service (NHS) hospitals in England.

Chapter 13

RISK FACTORS FOR CA-MRSA

Community-onset infection has been defined as an MRSA-positive culture of a sample obtained from an outpatient or from an inpatient within 48 h of admission. CA-MRSA infection has been defined by a community-onset infection in the absence of the health care-associated risk factors described above.

It is evident that skin integrity is important in the prevention of *S. aureus* infections. Many patients with CA-MRSA will report a breach in skin integrity that may serve as the portal for infection (Begier *et al.*, 2004; Kazakova *et al.*, 2005).

It is estimated that CA-MRSA colonizes about 3% of healthy individuals and could be a risk factor for the development of a CA-MRSA skin and soft tissue infection (Ellis *et al.*, 2004). Although the elimination of *S. aureus* nasal colonization with intranasal mupirocin in the hospital setting can reduce nosocomial infection (Perl *et al.*, 2002; von Eiff *et al.*, 2001), there are limited data showing that reducing CA-MRSA colonization decreases invasive disease. Data are emerging on the need to culture other anatomic sites besides the nares (ie, groin, rectum, and axillae) to obtain a true picture of CA-MRSA colonization (Rosenthal *et al.*, 2006).

Although many patients with CA-MRSA have no risk factors (Moran *et al.*, 2006), the factors associated with most high-risk groups include poor hygiene, overcrowded living conditions, skin-skin contact between individuals, sharing contaminated personal items, and trauma, all of which play a large role in disseminating organisms (Gorwitz *et al.*, 2008; Shastry *et al.*, 2007; Kazakova *et al.*, 2005; Turabelidze *et al.*, 2004). Many other risk factors have been found associated with CA-MRSA infection, such as prior health care exposure, incarceration, intravenous (IV) drug abuse, team sports, military training, and in men who have sex with men (Miller *et al.,* 2007; Kazakova *et al.,* 2005; Zinderman *et al.,*2004; Centers for Disease Control, 2003a, 2003b). However, more and more patients are presenting to the emergency department with CA-MRSA infection who have no identifiable risk factor (LoVecchio *et al.,* 2009).

Due to the ease of transmission from person to person or fomite to person, outbreaks of CA-MRSA SSTI are typically seen in populations with close contact (Shastry *et al.,* 2007; Kazakova *et al.,* 2005; Campbell *et al.,* 2004; Centers for Disease Control, 2001).

Specifically among competitive sports, the following risk factors have been identified: athletic teammates who are colonized (Kazovaza *et al.,* 2005), skin trauma (eg, turf burns, lacerations, abrasions), lineman or linebacker position on football teams, higher body mass index, cosmetic body shaving, physical contact with a person who has a draining lesion, and sharing equipment that is not cleaned or laundered between users (shared towels, razors, whirlpools, bars of soap). A lack of personal hygiene and a lack of basic infection-control principles probably contributed to these outbreaks (Miller & Diep, 2008; Begier *et al.,* 2004).

Outbreaks have occurred in athletes engaged in contact sports, including wrestlers, football players, rugby players, and fencers (Begier *et al.,* 2004; Kazovaza *et al.,* 2005; Centers for Diseasae Control, 2004), men who have sex with men (Diep *et al.,* 2008), prison inmates (Aiello *et al.,* 2006), children in daycare centers (Adcock *et al.,* 1998), and homeless individuals (Gilbert *et al.,* 2006). Other groups have been identified, such as closed religious groups, users of crystal methamphetamine, tattoo recipients (Centers for Diseasae Control, 2006), evacuees from Hurricane Katrina (Centers for Diseasae Control, 2005), and military personnel (Aiello *et al.,* 2006; Campbell *et al.,* 2004).

The risk factors identified in these outbreaks have reflected the conditions found in other CA-MRSA-outbreak settings and include close contact, compromised skin integrity, and limited access to adequate hygiene (Lowy *et al.,* 2007). It is estimated that more than 60% of households of children hospitalized with CA-MRSA infections have family members with a history of MRSA infection in the previous 6 months (Daum, 2007).

MRSA-outbreak investigations and cross-sectional studies of inmates in correctional facilities have identified some significant demographic risk factors, including comorbidities, female sex (for staphylococcal colonization), and longer incarceration. Similar to the men colonized with MSSA, those colonized with MRSA reported a higher incidence of fair/poor health and history of abscess. Additional factors associated specifically with MRSA colonization included reports of chronic skin disease, antibiotic use in the last 6 months, current abscess at the time of arrest, and active intravenous drug use in the last 6 months. Men colonized with MRSA but without a history of previous arrest maintained the same exact risk factors noted earlier (ie, history of abscess and age 30 to 49 years). Men with a history of previous arrest also were noted to have several additional risk factors, 2 of which were directly associated with previous incarceration activities: hospital admission within 6 months of arrest, skin infection during previous incarceration, and use of prison weight room/gym during previous incarceration (Farley *et al.*, 2008).

Populations most commonly infected by CA-MRSA include:

- Young children (Fridkin *et al.*, 2005)
- Daycare attendees (Adcock *et al.*, 1998)
- Prison inmates (Aiello *et al.*, 2006; Gilbert *et al.*, 2006)
- Indigenous populations (Centers for Diseasae Control, 2004; Groom *et al.*, 2001)
- Men who have sex with men (Diep *et al.*, 2008)
- HIV infection (Fridkin *et al.*, 2005)
- Members of football teams (Begier *et al.*, 2004; Kazovaza *et al.*, 2005; Centers for Diseasae Control, 2004)
- Wrestlers (Centers for Diseasae Control, 2003a)
- Fencing teams (Centers for Diseasae Control, 2003a)
- Injection drug users (Gilbert *et al.*, 2006)
- Homeless (Gilbert *et al.*, 2006)
- Tattoo recipients (Centers for Diseasae Control, 2006)
- Military recruits (Aiello *et al.*, 2006; Campbell *et al.*, 2004)

Chapter 14

PREVENTION

According to the Centers for Diseasae Control, CA-MRSA skin and soft tissue infection prevention lies in the "Five C's of CA-MRSA Transmission": contact, cleanliness, compromised skin, contaminated objects, and crowded conditions (Minnesota Department of Health, 2004).

To avoid infection, patients should be encouraged to avoid skin-to-skin contact, focus on good personal hygiene, avoid sharing personal items (Turabelidze *et al.*, 2004), limit activity that causes skin abrasions such as avoiding insect bites and body shaving, maintain as much environmental hygiene as possible, and avoid overcrowding (Minnesota Department of Health, 2004). Of note, currently, eliminating skin or nasal CA-MRSA colonization is not mentioned as the sixth C as carriage may play a much less prominent role in the pathogenesis of CA-MRSA than initially thought.

Given the rapidly growing epidemic in the community, at this point just about everyone is at risk. Risk reduction is probably best achieved through good hygiene. As skin-skin and skin-fomite contact are important routes of CA-MRSA acquisition, measures to limit its spread focus on wound coverage, hand washing, laundering of clothes, linens, and towels, and environmental decontamination, as recommended by an expert panel from the Centers for Disease Control and Prevention (Gorwitz *et al.*, 2008). For individuals with a recurrent MRSA infection, it is reasonable to attempt decolonization if standard prevention measures have failed (Gorwitz *et al.*, 2008). Decolonization regimens vary, but usually include the application of topical mupirocin ointment to the anterior nares twice daily for 5 days along with adjunctive chlorhexidine baths, using either 4% chlorhexidine gluconate-containing soap or 2% chlorhexidine gluconate wipes.

Several studies on *S. aureus*, suggest that MRSA infection usually follows prior carriage rather than occurring from direct transmission during invasive procedures by staff or from the ICU environment (von Eiff *et al.*, 2001; Chang *et al.*, 1998) meaning that MRSA infection is preceded by colonization with an MRSA strain that is genetically indistinguishable from the disease-causing isolate in at least 56% of patients. These data support the view that prevention of colonization of ICU patients with MRSA could reduce the frequency of MRSA infections (Keshtgar *et al.*, 2008) and can assist in the design of effective prevention strategies against MRSA infection (Khandavilli *et al.*, 2008).

Infection control for HA-MRSA focuses on hand hygiene, identification and contact isolation of MRSA carriers, patient decolonization, and environmental decontamination. Hand hygiene is likely the most important component of prevention and control of MRSA in the hospital. HA-MRSA is most commonly transmitted on the hands of health care workers (Pittet *et al.*, 2001). APIC recommends hand washing as a simple measure to prevent the spread of MRSA within medical institutions. A number of studies have shown that many health care workers are not appropriately vigilant about washing their hands consistently although hand hygiene is the most important means of preventing the spread of infection.

Universal MRSA screening of patients admitted to hospital is receiving an increasing amount of interest. In the USA, the introduction of universal admission MRSA screening in a three-hospital organization was associated with a drastic reduction of hospital-acquired MRSA infection within two years. However, an extensive review of the clinical and cost effectiveness of screening for MRSA in 2007 in Scotland concluded that there is still a lack of robust data to populate the economic model, and that the impact of screening strategies on the prevalence of MRSA in NHS hospitals cannot be reliably predicted. The use of decolonization therapy is controversial but may be warranted in individuals with multiple recurrences or in ongoing transmission within closely associated groups.

There is also controversy over whether active surveillance cultures prevent MRSA transmission or infections and whether these active surveillance cultures should be performed on all hospitalized patients. In one study, universal screening cultures on admission and weekly thereafter decreased the mean number of MRSA bacteremia cases from 3.6 to 1.8 cases per month (Shitrit *et al.*, 2006). This has also been suggested by other investigators (McGinigle *et al.*, 2008).

Contact isolation of MRSA carriers also prevents transmission within the hospital. These measures include: private room or cohorting in a room and using gown and non-sterile gloves for any anticipated contact with the patient or potentially contaminated areas in the patient's environment (Siegel *et al.,* 2007).

An important component of control of HA-MRSA is environmental decontamination. Investigators report rates as high as 53% of acquisition of MRSA on hands after contacting environmental surfaces near patients (Bhalla *et al.,* 2004).

According to the CDC, the survival of *S. aureus* and MRSA on environmental surfaces can range from few hours to several months depending on factors such as temperature, humidity, the bacterial load, and the type of surface (porous or nonporous). It also depends on whether these surfaces have nutrients to allow bacteria to survive longer. Un-cleaned surfaces naturally more likely support longer bacterial survival especially if accompanied by other favoring conditions. Covering cuts and wounds with bandages is important to avoid both contaminating the environment and getting infected even if contact occurs with contaminated surfaces.

The following is an example of how the public could be addressed to increase their awareness of measures to prevent spreading of MRSA:

Basic Steps for Prevention: Reduce the risk of spreading staph, including MRSA to others by following these steps:

- Keep uninfected cuts/wounds clean and covered; watch for signs of infection, such as redness, warmth, and swelling. If a sore or cut becomes red, oozes, causes pain, or isn't healing, see a doctor.
- Cover wounds. Pus from infected wounds can contain staph. Cover wounds that are draining or have pus with clean, dry bandages. Follow your healthcare provider's instructions on proper care of the wound. Bandages or tape can be discarded with the regular trash.
- Keep hands clean. Wash bare hands regularly and frequently with soap and warm water, especially after changing a bandage or touching an infected wound (even if gloves are worn). Alcohol-based hand sanitizers may be used if hands are not visibly soiled.
- Do not share personal items. Avoid sharing personal items such as towels, washcloths, razors, clothing, or uniforms. Wash soiled sheets, towels, and clothes with warm/hot water and laundry detergent. Drying clothes in a hot dryer, rather than air-drying, also helps kill bacteria in clothes.

- Use a barrier like clothing or towels between you and any surfaces you share with others (like gym equipment), and shower immediately after activities that involve direct skin contact with others.
- Keep the environment clean. Regularly clean frequently touched surfaces and other items that come into direct contact with infected skin.
- In gyms, locker rooms, and other places where many people come and go, repair or throw out equipment and furniture with damaged surfaces that cannot be thoroughly cleaned.
- Talk to your doctor. Tell any healthcare providers who treat you if you have had a MRSA infection.
- If prescribed antibiotics, take all the pills, even if you feel better before they are all gone. Don't insist on antibiotics for treating colds or other virus infections.

Antistaphylococcal immunization is an area of ongoing research. A *S. aureus* capsular polysaccharides vaccine conferred protective immunity in patients receiving hemodialysis; however, it did not show long-term efficacy in a phase III trial (Shinefield *et al.,* 2002).

Chapter 15

TREATMENT OF METHICILLIN RESISTANT *STAPHYLOCOCCUS AUREUS*

The very essence of classifying a *Staphylococcus aureus* isolate as methicillin resistant *Staphylococcus aureus* (MRSA) lies in its resistance to methicillin, a semisynthetic penicillin. However, this is not the only drug to which it is resistant. It actually has the machinery to defy all β-lactam antibiotics, such as penicillins and cephalosporins and carbapenems. MRSA's resistance to all forms of penicillin has earned it the moniker of "superbug." Due to its drug resistance, it is twice as fatal as other staph infections (Cosgrove *et al.*, 2003; Whitby *et al.*, 2001).

It has been contended that the introduction of methicillin put an end to the tremendous amount of research and enthusiasm for the infection control measures which were effective and vigorous at the time when it was first introduced. The medical community experienced a false sense of security against these resistant pathogens. Once you could treat these previously antibiotic-resistant staphylococci, people stopped washing their hands and doing all the other things they now realize they should have been doing all along.

MRSA, like other multidrug resistant organisms (MDR) really seem to be gathering pace, no doubt fuelled by intensive broad-spectrum antibiotic use, poor infection control, highly immunosuppressed patients, and rapid and frequent air travel.

Antibiotic resistance has reached crisis point in many hospitals around the world. Most are swamped with MRSA and many with MDR Gram-negative bacteria. Despite the availability of good treatment alternatives available for serious infections due to MRSA, mortality rates remain high.

Hospital acquired MRSA (HA-MRSA) has traditionally been resistant to other anti-staphylococcal agents, such as clindamycin, erythromycin, and tetracycline, with variable resistance to gentamicin and trimethoprim-sulfamethoxazole (SXT) whereas community-associated MRSA (CA-MRSA) isolates have typically been susceptible to clindamycin, SXT, and gentamicin.

Several studies from the USA have described the need for using empirical MRSA coverage in patients attending emergency departments.

It is imperative that clinicians have a high index of suspicion for MRSA so they can promptly initiate the appropriate antibiotic therapy. Failure to act quickly can lead to increased morbidity and mortality for patients. As more virulent strains and increasing resistance occur due to the dynamic nature of this pathogen, not only is the prevalence of CA-MRSA increasing, but the devastating mortality of these infections continue to be evident since the 4 pediatric deaths from CA-MRSA were reported in 1999 (CDC, 1999).

However, the decision of when to start systemic treatment can be difficult. Features such as fever, underlying illness such as diabetes mellitus, human immunodeficiency virus (HIV) or involvement of deep structures or extensive lesions or if there are infections in other family members support the use of systemic therapy (Enoch *et al.*, 2008).

ANTIBIOTIC DRUG DEVELOPMENT

Despite the continuing emergence of resistant pathogens, development of new classes of antimicrobials has been at a virtual standstill since the late 1970s (Spellberg *et al.*, 2004; IDSA, 2004) probably due to relatively unfavourable returns on investment. Four new classes of antibiotics were introduced in the 1930s and 1940s, including sulphonamides, β-lactams, aminoglycosides, and chloramphenicol. A further six classes were developed and approved in the 1950s and 1960s, including tetracycline, macrolides, glycopeptides, rifamycins, quinolones, and trimethoprim. However, from 1970 to the late 1990s, no new antimicrobial classes were approved and only a few new classes have been approved since 2000 for the treatment of Gram-positive infections; these are the oxazolidinones (linezolid), cyclic lipopeptides (daptomycin), and glycylcyclines (tigecycline). Pharmaceutical companies are discouraged from research and development of new antimicrobials due to high direct costs, risk, and the time associated with animal and in vitro studies

(Wenzel, 2004). There are already concerns about resistance to the 2 recently introduced antibiotics in the lipopeptide and oxazolidinone classes. Several reports have described cases of clinically significant resistance to daptomycin (a lipopeptide) for the treatment of MRSA infections (Hayden *et al.*, 2005; Mangili *et al.*, 2005; Vikram *et al.*, 2005), and there are currently 7 case reports of resistance to linezolid (an oxazolidinone) among individuals with *S. aureus* infections (Peters & Sarria, 2005).

Increasing levels of antibiotic resistance, the waning drug development pipeline, and declining numbers of pharmaceutical companies involved with the development of anti-infective agents create a significant public health threat to the effective management of bacterial infections (Wenzel, 2004). Additional factors (Rice, 2003) that establish the imperative for the development of new antibiotics include:

(1) Emergence of bacterial species resistant to new antibiotics.
(2) Intolerance to, or safety concerns about, treatment with currently available antibiotics, such as an increased risk of bleeding associated with linezolid.
(3) Current dosing regimens for most available antimicrobials that are incompatible with outpatient administration, resulting in prolonged hospital stay, increased cost, and increased exposure to nosocomial infections.

TREATMENT OF MRSA INFECTIONS

Vancomycin is currently the first-line agent for treating invasive MRSA infections. Glycopeptide antibiotics, which include vancomycin and teicoplanin, inhibit bacterial cell-wall synthesis. Vancomycin was developed more than 50 years ago and has been the mainstay of treatment for a variety of infections, including endocarditis, pneumonia, and wound infections, with cure rates estimated at 63%, 75%, and 90% of patients, respectively (Esposito & Gleckman, 1977). More recently, however, this role as mainstay of MRSA treatment has been called into question, in part because vancomycin has poorer tissue penetration, especially reported for lung tissue (Rybak, 2006; Cruciani *et al.*, 1996; Lamer *et al.*, 1993) and is less bactericidal with slower bacterial clearance than the anti-staphylococcal penicillins (Gould, 2007a; Chang *et al.*, 2003), it demonstrates poor pharmacokinetic properties, and fluctuating minimum inhibitory concentrations (MICs). Vancomycin monotherapy has demonstrated inferiority to beta-lactam therapy in the treatment of methicillin sensitive *S. aureus* osteomyelitis (Martinez-Aguilar *et al.,* 2003) and bacteraemia (Gould, 2007b; Stryjewski *et al.,* 2007; Siegman-Igra *et al.,* 2005; Chang *et al.,* 2003). Poor pharmacokinetic properties undermining the efficacy of vancomycin include variable tissue penetration and high inoculum sizes (Kollef, 2007; Stevens, 2006).

In a prospective study, 19% (13/70) of MSSA bacteraemia patients treated with vancomycin experienced bacteriological failure, with bacteraemia persisting beyond 7 days or with relapse, compared with none of 18 treated with nafcillin (Chang *et al.,* 2003). Similarly, none of ten patients treated with cloxacillin for MSSA pneumonia died, compared with 47% (8 / 17) of those treated with vancomycin (Gonzalez *et al.,*1999). So generally speaking, there is wide consensus that β-lactams are more efficacious than vancomycin against infections due to susceptible staphylococci.

Vancomycin is also associated with several other limitations, including the development of resistance and associated therapeutic failure, and the potential for serious toxicity. There is growing evidence of vancomycin resistance, including vancomycin-intermediate *S. aureus* (VISA) and heterogeneous VISA (hVISA), in patients with serious infections. hVISA is regarded as a precursor to VISA (Liu & Chambers, 2003): it comprises a heterogeneous population of *S. aureus* cells with an overall MIC in the susceptible range (i.e. < 2 μg/ml), but with non-susceptible subpopulations (i.e. with an overall MIC ≥4 μg/ml) detectable after selection with vancomycin. Heterogeneous VISA infections are associated with high treatment failure rates, prolonged bacteraemia, high bacterial loads, and lower vancomycin trough levels (Kollef, 2007; Stevens, 2006).

An additional concern about vancomycin includes adverse reactions, especially nephrotoxicity, when combined with aminoglycoside agents (Jeffres *et al.,* 2007). Vancomycin has also been shown to provoke hypersensitivity reactions, including anaphylaxis and 'red man syndrome' (an infusion-related reaction involving pruritus and an erythematous rash) (Kollef, 2007).

The standard treatment options for serious MRSA infections are the glycopeptides, vancomycin and teicoplanin, often given together with rifampicin. According to the susceptibility of the particular strain, combinations of two or more of fusidic acid, rifampicin, trimethoprim and minocycline may also be used in less severe infections or as oral follow-on treatment to an intravenous glycopeptide. In addition, there is a growing list of recently developed agents for treatment of severe MRSA infection, with quinupristin–dalfopristin, daptomycin, linezolid and tigecycline already licensed in some parts of the world, and dalbavancin and telavancin anticipated in the next few years (Abbanat *et al.*, 2003; Anstead & Owens, 2004). However, all of these agents are significantly more expensive than the older oral agents, and all but linezolid require intravenous administration.

The SENTRY surveillance program (SENTRY is an international antimicrobial surveillance program that documents resistance patterns in bacteria isolated from predominantly hospitalized patients) revealed *S. aureus* to be the leading cause of skin and soft-tissue infections (SSTIs), and the second most common causative organism for bacteraemia in Europe (Moet *et al.*, 2007; Biedenbach *et al.*, 2004). MRSA is of particular concern, as it is associated with greater mortality than MSSA (Cosgrove *et al.*, 2003; Whitby *et al.*, 2001). Although vancomycin is the most widely used agent against Gram positive infections, against *S. aureus*, other agents have demonstrated equivalent and/or superior efficacy to vancomycin in clinical trials of MRSA and MSSA infections (Rehm et al. 2008; Stryjewski *et al.*, 2007; Weigelt *et al.*, 2005; Arbeit *et al.*, 2004; Chang *et al.*, 2003; Stevens *et al.*, 2002; Gentry *et al.*, 1997).

For the treatment of complicated skin and soft tissue infections (cSSTIs), daptomycin showed equivalent efficacy to standard therapy, which comprised vancomycin for suspected MRSA infections and required shorter duration of therapy (Whitby *et al.*, 2001). Daptomycin is a cyclic lipopeptide that depolarizes the bacterial cell membrane. It is a fermentation product of *Streptomyces roseosporus* consisting of a 13-member amino acid cyclic lipopeptide with a decanoyl side chain (Enoch *et al.*, 2008; Micek, 2007). Daptomycin was approved by the United States Food and Drug Administration (USA-FDA) and by the European Medicines Agency (EMEA) for the treatment of cSSSIs caused by methicillin-susceptible and methicillin-resistant *S. aureus*, Daptomycin has shown equivalent efficacy to vancomycin against MRSA bacteraemia/infective endocarditis and might provide an alternative treatment option (Rehm *et al.*, 2008). Although these compounds (daptomycin, linezolid, vancomycin) show similar susceptibility rates, daptomycin was four- to eightfold more active than vancomycin or linezolid (Sader *et al.*, 2009).

Daptomycin is also as effective as standard therapy against MSSA bacteraemia/infective endocarditis (Fowler *et al.*, 2006). In the majority of relevant case reports, daptomycin was administered when treatment of patients with endocarditis or bacteraemia with other potentially effective antibiotics (including glycopeptides and linezolid) had failed (Falagas et al, 2007).

Because of its excellent anti-*S. aureus* spectrum, high potency, and rapid bactericidal activity, daptomycin represents an excellent treatment option for

BSI caused by *S. aureus* in at-risk patients such as those on hemodialysis (Sader *et al.*, 2009). In fact, it is the only new antibiotic with a license for use in staphylococcal blood stream infections (Rose *et al.*, 2008). An antibiotic that has high clinical efficacy against both MSSA and MRSA infections is of particular value as an alternative to vancomycin, given that suspected *S. aureus* infections are often treated empirically and the consequences of inappropriate antimicrobial use, such as vancomycin for an infection later confirmed to be MSSA, can be severe (Gould, 2008). Daptomycin does not exhibit cross-resistance with other known classes of antimicrobials and also has a low risk for development of spontaneous mutational resistance (Sader *et al.*, 2009). Resistance to daptomycin remains low although it should always be checked for if there has been prior glycopeptide exposure in a patient (Rose *et al.*, 2008). Indeed, daptomycin has been shown to be active against methicillin resistant *S. aureus* (MRSA) as well as *S. aureus* resistant to linezolid or quinupristin/dalfopristin (Sader *et al.*, 2009).

Linezolid is a synthetic oxazolidinone that inhibits bacterial protein synthesis by binding to the bacterial 23S ribosomal RNA of the 50S subunit. The antibiotic is bacteriostatic against staphylococci. Linezolid received US Food and Drug Administration approval in 2000 and has demonstrated clinical success against indicated Gram-positive organisms causing a variety of infections including serious cutaneous disease and nosocomial pneumonia (Weigelt *et al.*, 2005; Wunderink *et al.*, 2003; Stevens *et al.*, 2002). It is currently approved for the treatment of complicated skin and skin-structure infections (SSSIs) and nosocomial pneumonia caused by MRSA (Vergidis & Falagas, 2008). For the treatment of SSTIs caused by MRSA, linezolid has shown equivalent or greater efficacy to vancomycin in a number of trials (Weigelt *et al.*, 2005; Stevens *et al.*, 2002) and required a shorter duration of hospital stay for complicated SSTIs (Li *et al.*, 2003). There is limited evidence, based on subset analysis, to suggest that linezolid is superior to vancomycin in treating nosocomial pneumonia due to MRSA (Wunderink *et al.*, 2003). Resistance to linezolid remains very uncommon (<0.5%) among surveyed isolates. However, with wider linezolid use, resistance has been recognized (Baddour *et al.*, 2006; Gales *et al.*, 2006; Mutnick *et al.*, 2003; Jones *et al.*, 2002; Marshall *et al.*, 2002; Gonzales *et al.*, 2001; Tsiodras *et al.*, 2001) and characterized as associated with prolonged drug exposure in at-risk patient populations or with breaks in infection control practices (Kainer *et al.*, 2007; Mutnick *et al.*, 2003). Treatment failure typically occurs as a result of deep infection and failure to drain abscesses (Enoch *et al.*, 2008).

Dalfopristin is a derivative of a group A streptogramin, and quinupristin is a group B streptogramin. The streptogramins are a family of compounds isolated from *Streptomyces pristinaespiralis*. These 2 water-soluble streptogramins have been combined in a commercially available injectable form at a 30:70 weight-to-weight ratio (Allington & Rivey, 2001). Individually, quinupristin and dalfopristin demonstrate only modest in vitro bacteriostatic activity. However, the combination of the 2 commonly produces in vitro bactericidal activity that is 8 to 16 times higher than the sum of each component's activity against many gram-positive organisms (Aeschlimann & Rybak, 1998; Rubinstein & Bompart, 1997; Caron et al, 1997). Quinupristin and dalfopristin bind to sequential sites located on the 50s subunit of the bacterial ribosome. Dalfopristin binding causes a conformational change in the ribosome that subsequently increases the binding of quinupristin. The combined actions of the 2 agents create a stable drug-ribosome complex that causes inhibition of protein synthesis by several mechanisms, including prevention of peptide-chain formation, blockade of extrusion of newly formed peptide chains, and, in many instances, bacterial cell death (Thal & Zervos, 1999). Streptogramin resistance is mediated by 3 possible mechanisms: drug inactivation by enzymes, efflux or active transport of the antibiotic out of the cell, and conformational alterations in ribosomal target binding sites. The latter is the most common expression of bacterial resistance to streptogramins. Quinupristin/dalfopristin is active against *S. aureus*, including MRSA, and has been approvedby the FDA for treatment of Gram-positive bacteraemia.

Tigecycline, the first of a new synthetic class of antibiotics known as glycylcyclines, was approved in 2005 (Pankey, 2005). It is a derivative of minocycline and acts by inhibiting the 30S ribosomal subunit and thus protein synthesis. Tigecycline was developed to overcome tetracycline resistance mediated by efflux pumps and ribosomal protection. Tigecycline is a broad-spectrum antibiotic with activity against gram-positive, gram-negative, and atypical anaerobes (Nathwani, 2005). In a multicentre study across Europe testing for comparative antimicrobial susceptibility, tigecycline was the only agent to which all Gram-positive isolates were susceptible (Rodloff *et al.,*2008). Gram-positive bacteria that are susceptible to tigecycline include MRSA, glycopeptide-intermediate *S. aureus* (GISA), vancomycin-resistant enterococci (Cercenado *et al.*, 2003; Petersen *et al.*, 2002) and penicillin-resistant *Streptococcus pneumoniae* (Hoellman *et al.*, 2000). In June 2005, the drug was approved by the FDA for treatment of complicated SSSIs, including those caused by MSSA and MRSA.

Chapter 16

TREATMENT OF CA-MRSA

Based on the escalating observance of CA-MRSA in different settings, it has been proposed that CA-MRSA is going to become one of the most challenging infectious disease problems in the 21st century (Deurenberg *et al.,* 2007; Vandenesch *et al.,* 2003).

Physicians evaluating patients with skin and soft tissue infections in the outpatient and emergency departments must be cognizant of the likelihood that CAMRSA is the offending organism. The paradigm that simple abscesses without cellulitis (focal skin/soft tissue infections), require only incision and drainage has not changed (LoVecchio *et al.,* 2009; Ruhe et al., 2007; Martinez-Aguilar et al., 2003).

Clinicians should be aware that the prevalence of CA-MRSA has increased markedly over the past few years. The virulence of these new strains of CA-MRSA is unique not only in the resistance to β-lactam antibiotics but in their capacity to cause tissue necrosis. When approaching a patient with a SSTI, clinicians are required to have a low threshold for sending material for culture and susceptibility testing when an incision and drainage is required. Empiric treatment of a SSTI should take into consideration providing coverage for CA-MRSA, MSSA, and *S. pyogenes* until an organism can be identified through culture. Clinicians should also be aware that, in the empiric selection of antibiotics, trimethoprim-sulfamethoxazole does not adequately cover *S. pyogenes.* Finally, in the setting of more invasive SSTI (pyomyositis or necrotizing fasciitis), empiric intravenous antibiotics directed against CA-MRSA must be included in the initial treatment regimen. There are surprisingly few data regarding oral treatment of the common and serious problem of SSTI caused by MRSA. A case can certainly be made for treating simple and uncomplicated skin infections with surgical drainage alone and reserving the use of systemic antibiotics for patients with fever, large abscesses, complications or underlying risk factors. Drainage of abscesses is required even if antibiotics are used. The latest British Society for Antimicrobial Chemotherapy (BSAC) guideline advises against giving systemic antibiotics to patients with minor SSTIs or small abscesses <5 cm. Thus small abscesses without cellulitis should be incised and drained and antibiotics withheld (Nathwani *et al.,* 2008).

Recent literature has suggested different approaches to the treatment of skin and soft tissue infections. Localized skin infections, including small furuncles and abscesses, often respond to surgical incision and drainage alone, but nonetheless, oral antimicrobials are commonly prescribed. For large soft tissue infection with surrounding cellulitis, lacking a drainable focus, and with systemic symptoms such as fever, most physicians would treat with antimicrobial drugs, although controlled trials are lacking (Moellering RC Jr, 2008; Gorwitz, 2007). Such infections include cellulitis, osteomyelitis, diabetic foot infections, and urinary tract infections [UTIs]). Many such infections receive extended treatment, often in the outpatient setting, which makes intravenous therapy unattractive. Selection of appropriate antibiotics for MRSA infection depends on several factors, including severity of disease (local versus invasive) and strain of MRSA.

Although some reports claim there is no difference between the outcome of septic arthritis caused by MSSA and MRSA (Al-Nammari *et al.,*2007), evidence from other reports show that septic arthritis caused by CA-MRSA could be associated with more severe outcome (Castaldo and Yang, 2007; Arnold *et al.,*2006). In fact, the 1st genome of CA-MRSA sequenced was from a strain that caused fatal septicemia and septic arthritis (Baba *et al.,*2002).

Current guidelines recommend broad-spectrum combination therapy with more than 2 antibiotics as the initial empirical therapy for some types of infections in patients at risk of being infected with resistant organisms (American Thoracic Society, IDSA, 2005). All antibiotics can potentially exert selective pressure and thereby drive resistance Deresinski, 2007b), yet appropriate empiric antimicrobial therapy is important because it can decrease mortality in critically ill patients (Kumar *et al.,* 2006; Ibrahim *et al.,* 2000; Kollef, 2000).

CA-MRSA strains differ in antimicrobial susceptibility compared with hospital-acquired MRSA, because CA-MRSA strains often lack resistance to several various non-ß-lactam antibiotics, a feature most likely attributable to a lower frequency of antibiotic-selective pressures in the community compared with the hospital environment (Chambers, 2001; Suggs *et al.,* 1999). However, with the migration of CA-MRSA strains into hospital settings and movement of these strains back out to the community, an agile CA-MRSA strain with multidrug resistance traits may emerge (Carleton *et al.,* 2004).

Oral agents such as SXT, clindamycin, doxycyline, linezolid, rifampin, and occasionally fluoroquinolones have been used for minor skin infections. In the United States, current susceptibility patterns suggest that all CAMRSA isolates are susceptible to SXT and rifampin, 95% are susceptible to clindamycin, 92% are susceptible to tetracycline, 60% are susceptible to fluoroquinolones, and 6% are susceptible to erythromycin (Moran *et al.,* 2006). But which drug is the first choice, what the regimen should be and whether it should be used in combination are currently more art than science.

In addition to vancomycin, newer parenteral agents for more severe invasive infections include linezolid, daptomycin, and tigecycline; additional potential treatment options are in development.

Chapter 17

TREATMENT OF VISA AND VRSA

Reduced susceptibility of *S. aureus* to vancomycin and teicoplanin has been definitively observed in recent years with the emergence of glycopeptide-resistant *S. aureus* (GRSA), glycopeptide-intermediate *S. aureus* (GISA) and heterogeneous GISA (hGISA) (Pope & Roecker, 2007; Liu & Chambers, 2003). There is a growing body of evidence that shows the MICs of glycopeptides against *S. aureus* strains to be increasing incrementally, a process referred to as MIC creep.

The prevalence and clinical significance of hVISA cannot be accurately addressed. Furthermore, strains assayed prior to the introduction of reduced CLSI MIC breakpoints in 2006 would be subject to less stringent categorization than they would be today. It is clear from retrospective studies and testing of previously isolated strains that the presence of VISA and hVISA was overlooked prior to 1996. Also, with the variation in effectiveness of susceptibility tests used, and without consensus on how hVISA MICs should be measured, it is difficult to gauge the true extent of vancomycin resistance and reduced susceptibility today.

The *in vitro* activities of a number of antibiotic agents against VISA and hVISA strains have been examined, although the clinical efficacy of such agents has not yet been established in the published literature.

In the SENTRY surveillance program, lower MIC values were measured for daptomycin (0.12–2 µg/ml) compared with vancomycin (1–8 µg/ml) against hVISA and VISA, as well as vancomycin-susceptible MRSA and MSSA (Wootton *et al.,* 2006). In time–kill experiments in two GISA and one hGISA strain, daptomycin at 2 × MIC demonstrated bactericidal activity throughout the 24-hour measurement period and displayed 99.9% kill by 8 hours in all three strains (LaPlante & Rybak, 2004). Arbekacin and tigecycline also showed activity against these strains over 24 hours, whereas in contrast, vancomycin displayed no activity at the 24-hour timepoint.

There has been some concern that *S. aureus* strains with reduced susceptibility to vancomycin may also have reduced susceptibility to daptomycin. In the MIC surveillance study by Steinkraus *et al.* (Steinkraus *et al.*, 2007), daptomycin MICs did not increase over the 5-year period, despite vancomycin MICs incrementally increasing, suggesting that cross-resistance was not occurring. All VRSA strains identified to date have been found susceptible to daptomycin (Patel *et al.*, 2006), but a proportion of VISA isolates have shown reduced daptomycin susceptibility (Moise *et al.*, 2008; Cui *et al.*, 2006; Patel *et al.*, 2006; Sader *et al.*, 2006). Reduced susceptibility in some VISA strains may be a result of adaptive modifications such as thickened cell walls, reducing antibiotic penetration – other resistance mechanisms such as *vanA*-mediated resistance should not influence susceptibility to agents with a different mode of action to vancomycin. In a recent study of 81 patients with MRSA bacteraemia, prior vancomycin exposure within 30 days was associated with significantly higher vancomycin MICs and reduced vancomycin killing activity *in vitro* (Moise *et al.*, 2008). In contrast, there was only a trend towards higher daptomycin MICs with previous vancomycin exposure, and daptomycin retained its full *in vitro* bactericidal activity (Moise *et al.*, 2008). That previous vancomycin exposure does not affect a reduction in the bactericidal activity of daptomycin is supported by a separate study of VISA isolates (Sader *et al.*, 2006).

Other antibiotics have also shown activity in VISA and hVISA; in a comparison of eight licensed antibiotics, linezolid and quinupristin/dalfopristin were the only agents to demonstrate potent activity against VISA and hVISA. The MICs for linezolid were consistently low (0.25–2 μg/ml), whereas the MICs for quinupristin/dalfopristin were more variable (0.25–16 μg/ml) (Howe *et al.*, 2003).

Chapter 18

VANCOMYCIN TREATMENT FAILURES

MRSA infections can be difficult to treat. Clinical failures, even with appropriate treatment, occur regularly with vancomycin monotherapy, resulting in recommendations that vancomycin be used in combination with other antimicrobial agents to yield the best clinical results.

Appropriate treatment could be defined as intravenous treatment with an antibiotic to which the infecting bacterial strain is susceptible for at least 1 week in pneumonia, 2 weeks in bloodstream infections, 4 weeks in endocarditis, epidural abscess, and joint infection; and 6 weeks in osteomyelitis (Gilbert *et al.,* 2007). In cases of bloodstream infection, removal of intravascular catheters is considered a necessary part of appropriate treatment.

In 2006, increasing reports of vancomycin treatment failure and decreased susceptibility of MRSA to vancomycin prompted the Clinical and Laboratory Standards Institute (CLSI) to decrease the vancomycin breakpoint for *S. aureus* from 4 to 2 mg/L (Clinical and Laboratory Standards Institute, 2006).

Some clinical failures among MRSA infections treated with vancomycin may result from decreased susceptibility to the drug. MRSA strains with intermediate susceptibility to vancomycin (VISA; vancomycin minimum inhibitory concentration [MIC] = 4-8 µg/mL) and strains with frank resistance to vancomycin (VRSA; MIC $\geq$16 µ/mL) remain uncommon. However, some portion of vancomycin failures may be due to unrecognized heterogeneously resistant *S. aureus* (hVISA) (Liu & Chambers, 2003). Heteroresistance does not correlate well with MIC, and is thus not readily detected by standard clinical laboratory methods (Tenover & Moellering, 2007; Baddour *et al.,* 2007). Furthermore, infections due to MRSA which are still considered susceptible to vancomycin but have MICs at the higher end of the susceptible range (MIC=2) are at higher risk for clinical failure (Tenover & Moellering, 2007).

Years of glycopeptide under-dosing owing to fears of toxicity coupled with the poor penetration of glycopeptides into tissues (e.g. lung and endocardial tissue), is thought to have played a part in the emergence of reduced susceptibility by exposing *S. aureus* to sub-inhibitory concentrations of vancomycin (Deresinski, 2007a; Gould, 2007a; Sakoulas *et al.*, 2006). Glycopeptides are also only weakly bactericidal, and this might also have contributed to the development of strains with reduced susceptibility.

Interestingly, some studies claim that there was no association between patient outcomes and the susceptibility of the pathogen to the prescribed antimicrobial agents (Enoch *et al.*, 2008; Fridkin *et al.*, 2005; Lee *et al.*, 2004).

Apart from the intrinsic pharmacologic properties of vancomycin and emerging resistance, other factors may affect MRSA treatment failure rates. These include the site of infection, characteristics of the patient, antibiotic dosing and serum drug concentrations, and the presence and quality of concomitant surgical therapy where indicated. Such factors, however, are not well studied.

For MRSA bacteraemia/infective endocarditis, vancomycin is considered the gold-standard treatment. However, there have been recent reports of treatment failures against vancomycin-susceptible strains (Howden *et al.*, 2004; Charles *et al.*, 2004). In one study, glycopeptide therapy failed in 19/25 patients with infections caused by MRSA that conformed to definitions of VISA or hVISA by population analysis profiling (Howden *et al.*, 2004). In another prospective study, 19% (13/70) of MSSA bacteraemia patients treated with vancomycin experienced bacteriological failure, with bacteraemia persisting beyond 7 days or with relapse, compared with none of 18 treated with nafcillin (Chang *et al.*, 2003). Similarly, none of ten patients treated with cloxacillin for MSSA pneumonia died, compared with 47% (8/17) of those treated with vancomycin (Gonzalez *et al.*,1999). A separate study showed vancomycin treatment to fail in 5/5 MRSA patients with VISA, compared with 1/48 patients with vancomycin-susceptible MRSA (Charles *et al.*, 2004). Alternative treatments to vancomycin may be considered for the empiric therapy of suspected MRSA bacteraemia/infective endocarditis before the MIC and the presence of VISA or hVISA have been determined (Gould, 2008).

Another site of infection where this reported clinical failure occurs frequently despite appropriate therapy is the bones. Daver and colleagues recently reported a failure rate of 35% in patients with MRSA osteomyelitis treated with either ≥4 weeks of parenteral antibiotics or <4 weeks of parenteral therapy followed by oral therapy, with no difference in the relapse rates between the two groups (Daver *et al.*, 2007). Dombrowski and Winston, 2008, also reported a 25% clinical failure rate in an appropriately treated (Gilbert *et al.*, 2007) cohort of patients with diverse clinical conditions. They report that factors associated with an increased risk of failure at a *p*-value of <0.05 in bivariate analysis included diabetes, admission to the orthopedics service, osteomyelitis, and hospitalization in the intensive care unit at the time of antibiotic initiation. Pneumonia and endocarditis were associated with decreased risk of failure. In multivariate analysis, only a diagnosis of osteomyelitis was independently associated with failure ($p < 0.001$). They conclude justifiably that failure in cases of osteomyelitis was particularly common (46%) (Dombrowski and Winston, 2008).

It seems that regimens other than vancomycin monotherapy and/or longer duration of monotherapy may be more appropriate for treatment of MRSA osteomyelitis. In animal models of *S. aureus* osteomyelitis, vancomycin monotherapy has demonstrated inferiority to moxifloxacin (Kalteis et al, 2006), tigecycline (Yin et al, 2005), and rifampin-vancomycin combination therapy (Norden & Shaffer). Use of surgical debridement followed by local implantation of gatifloxacin implants had a favourable outcome in experimental MRSA osteomyelitis (ElKamel & Baddour, 2007).

The substantial failure rates in cases of MRSA osteomyelitis that are reported may also indicate poor performance of vancomycin in bone. Vancomycin has higher penetration into infected bone than non-infected bone, but it may function more poorly in the more anaerobic environment of osteomyelitic bone (Garazzino *et al.*, 2008).

The empirical use of vancomycin against Gram-positive infections should be carefully considered in the context of local vancomycin MIC data and, where possible, local MIC trends should be taken into account. Where vancomycin MIC is >1 μg/ml, alternative therapies should be considered to avoid the possibility of treatment failure. Precise determination of MIC, as well as regular surveillance are therefore of key importance because even small changes in MIC can have clinical significance (Gould, 2008).

Chapter 19

TREATMENT OPTIONS AND
NEW DIRECTIONS

MRSA are inherently resistant to all β-lactam antibiotics, but some lineages (clones) have additionally evolved resistance to multiple antibiotic classes. Within the species, resistance to all known antibiotic classes has occurred due to mutation and horizontal gene transfer and this has led to anxiety regarding the future availability of effective chemotherapeutic options.

Fortunately, most MRSA isolates remain susceptible to 1 or more of several older oral antimicrobial agents, including SXT, clindamycin, tetracyclines, and fluoroquinolones (Klevens et al., 2006; Moran et al., 2006).

Use of older oral agents could potentially slow the development of resistance to newer antimicrobials, avoid the morbidity and expense of intravenous access, and reduce drug costs.

This has prompted interest in such compounds for oral therapy for non-life-threatening MRSA infections (Stevens *et al.,* 2005). However, studies examining tetracycline (Ruhe and Menon, 2007; Ruhe *et al.,* 2005; Yuk *et al.,* 1991), SXT (Cenizal *et al.,* 2007; Markowitz *et al.,* 1992), or clindamycin (Martinez-Aguilar *et al.,* 2003) for treating MRSA infections were relatively small, involved only intravenous therapy, and/or were limited to a single type of infection.

In a study assessing the efficacy of alternative older antibiotics against MRSA, treatment was clinically successful in 89% of cases. The most commonly used alternative agent was SXT (49%), followed by long-acting tetracyclines (doxycycline and minocycline, 35%). SXT has received comparatively little attention in this role, and the attention it has received includes cautionary comments regarding the paucity of clinical data. Although Markowitz et al. (1992) showed good efficacy with intravenous SXT for serious MRSA infections (including bacteremia and endocarditis), evidence supporting oral SXT therapy for MRSA infections is quite limited (Stein et al., 1998; Honda et al., 1996). This has been the subject of a recent review by Proctor, who states that the new strains of community-acquired MRSA show decreased resistance to SXT. Clinical and experimental reports show a mixture of successes and failures with SXT. A reason for failure might be the amount of thymidine released from damaged host tissues and bacteria, a concept strengthened by the fact that *S. aureus* thermonuclease releases thymidine from DNA. Thus, success or failure with SXT may well depend on the amount of tissue damage and organism burden, rather than acquisition of a resistance gene. Clinical trials and experimental animal studies show high failure rates, perhaps because of released thymidine. He concludes that the use of SXT for community-acquired MRSA infection should not be endorsed without further research (Proctor, 2008).

A more recent retrospective assessment of alternative (non-vancomycin, non-linezolid) oral antimicrobial therapy for non-life-threatening MRSA infections for a 2-year period at a Veterans Affairs Medical Center demonstrated that this strategy was generally successful and well tolerated. Nearly 90% of subjects had satisfactory outcomes, and nearly half (40%) of the failures resulted from medication intolerance rather than frank clinical failure (Drekonja *et al.*, 2009).

There are several new classes with activity against MRSA which are currently in development. New glycopeptide agents include dalbavancin and telavancin, which are suitable for the treatment of MRSA and VISA strains and exhibit activity against a variety of other organisms (Billeter *et al.*, 2008; Jauregui *et al.*, 2005). Dalbavancin is a semi-synthetic lipoglycopeptide derived from a teicoplanin-like glycopeptide agent (Billeter *et al.*, 2008). It inhibits cell wall synthesis and has in vitro activity against MRSA with a long half-life of 6-10 d that allows once-weekly Dosing (Micek, 2007). Dalbavancin demonstrated similar cure rates when compared with linezolid for treating cSSTIs (Jauregui *et al.*, 2005). Dalbavancin seems to be a safe drug, with the most commonly reported adverse events including nausea, diarrhoea, and constipation with some evidence suggesting an increased risk of hypotension, hypokalemia, and increased levels of alanine aminotransferase and aspartate aminotransferase (Billeter *et al.*, 2008; Micek, 2007).

Telavancin is an investigational lipoglycopeptide antimicrobial agent with a dual mechanism of action that inhibits cell wall synthesis and disrupts membrane barrier function. Its half life ranges from 7 to 9 h, which permits once-daily dosing at 7.5 10 mg/kg/day. Disruption of the membrane barrier function permits rapid bactericidal activity for a variety of pathogens including MRSA and other drug-resistant strains. In vivo studies have demonstrated that telavancin may be effective for the treatment of Gram-positive soft tissue infections, bacteraemia, endocarditis, meningitis, and pneumonia. Furthermore, the MIC of telavancin is generally 2-8 times less than that of vancomycin for many Gram-positive bacteria, including MRSA (Attwood & LaPlante, 2007). Telavancin also appears to be more effective for the treatment of MRSA SSTIs infections than vancomycin (Stryjewski et al., 2006).

A major coming challenge will be to determine to what extent these agents offer absolute and cost-benefit advantages over vancomycin and to define their relative merits. The lack of wider evidence of superiority is perhaps surprising because vancomycin is not considered to be an especially potent antibiotic.

For severe clinical infections caused by MRSA, vancomycin remains the pivotal parenteral agent. However, numerous reports have confirmed the often slow and suboptimal treatment outcome when using vancomycin in single drug or combination therapy (Fowler et al., 1999; Levine et al., 1991). Thus, it seems essential to evaluate new antistaphylococcal drugs and regimens.

In principle, it should be possible to redesign β-lactams so that they bind to PBP2′, thereby gaining activity against MRSA. This task should be facilitated because the crystal structure of PBP2′ is known, permitting molecular modeling (Lim & Strynadka, 2002). Moreover, PBP2′ is exposed on the cell surface, meaning that the antibiotic need not be a good permeant of bacterial membranes, whereas this would be a sine qua non for an anti- Gram-negative agent. The problem lies in the fact that the active site of PBP2′ is located in an extended, narrow groove. The structure of this groove is such that the β-lactam is displaced and misaligned with respect to the active site serine residue, militating against acylation (Chambers, 2003; Lim & Strynadka, 2002). Many attempts have been made to produce β-lactams with modified side group structures to promote association with PBP2′ and to make acylation more energetically favourable. Modifications known to enhance activity involve acyl substituent groups with greater length and hydrophobicity, which result in increased interaction with the active site groove. Such research has yielded several compounds with MIC values of 2-8 mg/ L for MRSA (Chambers, 2003), but it has proved difficult to develop these for clinical use. One of the earliest such analogues, an aminothiazolylpenicillin called BRL-44154 (Beecham), was investigated in the 1980s (Mizen *et al.*, 1995) and had MICs of 4–8 mg/ L for MRSA, compared with 0.5–2 mg/ L for MSSA. It was effective against MRSA infections in mice but was inactivated by rapid metabolism in humans. A later carbapenem, L-695 256 (Merck), was even more active in vitro, with MICs of 2 mg/ L for MRSA, and was effective against MRSA endocarditis in rabbits (Chambers, 1995). However, it readily formed insoluble crystals, making it unsuitable for use in humans or for commercial manufacture (Sundelof *et al.*, 1996). Numerous anti-MRSA cephalosporins (e.g., TOC-50) (Nomura *et al.*, 1996) were presented at one or more ICAAC meetings during the 1990s before fading from view, usually without publicly available explanation. More recent anti-MRSA cephalosporins include RWJ-54428, now abandoned (Chamberland *et al.*, 2001), CAB-175 (Iizawa *et al.*, 2004; Koga *et al.*, 2005) and PPI-0903 (CX- 0903, T-91825, TAK-599) (Iizawa *et al.*, 2004), which is in phase I development, as is an anti-MRSA carbapenem, CS-023 (RO4908463) (Koga *et al.*, 2005).

One further promising anti-MRSA broad-spectrum cephalosporin, ceftobiprole (Ro 63-9141, BAL9141), has progressed much further. Ceftobiprole displays a wide range of activity both against Gram-positive and Gram-negative pathogens, including several resistant species such as MRSA, penicillin-resistant *Streptococcus pneumoniae* (Fritsche *et al.*, 2008; Rouse *et al.*, 2007; Jones *et al.*, 2002; Hebeisen *et al.*, 2001) and even heteroresistant vancomycin-intermediate *S. aureus* (hVISA) (MICs≤2mg/L) (Deshpande *et al.*, 2004). It is approved in Canada with the indication of cSSTIs. Ceftobiprole has an oxyimino aminothiazolyl substituent linked to the 7-amino group of the cephalosporin nucleus, conferring stability to many β-lactamases, and a vinylpyrrolidinone moiety at position 3, promoting association with PBP2' and facilitating the subsequent acylation reaction (Livermore, 2006). PBP assays, which reflect both the initial binding and the acylation, indicate that ceftobiprole produces a 50% saturation of PBP2' at an extremely low concentration compared with those needed for ceftriaxone, imipenem and methicillin (Hebeisen *et al.*, 2001). For improved solubility, ceftobiprole is administered in vivo as a water-soluble ester prodrug, ceftobiprole medocaril, which is rapidly cleaved in plasma to yield the active compound (Hebeisen *et al.*, 2001). The pharmacokinetics of ceftobiprole is similar to other β-lactams in that it displays a two-compartment model, distributes into extracellular fluid, does not cross membranes well and is primarily cleared renally. Ceftobiprole also displays a safety profile similar to other β-lactams, with the exception of dysgeusia being a common adverse effect. The potential for resistance development is low and therefore ceftobiprole seems to be good first-line therapeutic option against a variety of infections. This compound is not active against all pathogens and is subject to hydrolysis by some ESBLs and carbapenemases (Barbour *et al.*, 2009). It is currently under review by the FDA for approval in the USA.

Iclaprim is a selective dihydrofolate reductase inhibitor from a class of diaminopyrimidines that is currently in phase 3 trials. Iclaprim at concentrations close to the MIC has exhibited antimicrobial efficacy against Gram-positive pathogens including resistant *S. aureus* (MRSA, VISA, GISA) (Schneider *et al.*, 2003). The antibacterial profile of iclaprim compared with linezolid and vancomycin for treatment of SSTIs is promising (Morgan *et al.*, 2009).

Chapter 20

THE MICROBIOLOGY LABORATORY

In the microbiology laboratories, a few points have to be kept in mind, sometimes MRSA appears susceptible *in vitro* to other β-lactam agents, such as cephalosporins; however, these are not clinically effective. MRSA must be reported by the microbiology laboratory as resistant to all β-lactam agents (including cephalosporins, β-lactam and β-lactamase inhibitor combinations, and carbapenems), regardless of the *in vitro* test results.

Microbiology laboratories should also be aware that the results of testing for clindamycin susceptibility in CA-MRSA may be misleading. Treatment failures have been documented when MRSA isolates were reported as susceptible to clindamycin but resistant to erythromycin. A double-disk diffusion test (D zone test) should be performed to identify inducible clindamycin resistance in erythromycin resistant, clindamycin-susceptible *S. aureus* isolates (Yilmaz *et al.*, 2007).

Clinical microbiologists and infectious disease clinicians should be aware that staphylococci showing reduced susceptibility to vancomycin may also demonstrate reduced susceptibility to daptomycin. Such strains must be tested in the clinical microbiology laboratory for their susceptibility to daptomycin by a reliable and easy to use method. E-test strips are available and have been reported to give results comparable with the CLSI reference method (Fuchs *et al.*, 2001).

In conclusion, this growing threat of MRSA is becoming increasingly recognized by the public and health care providers. In 2008, MRSA has evolved to be commonplace in the community and hospital setting. MRSA infections are yet another major factor in the spiraling costs of health care (it is estimated that it costs $4–7 billion annually in the USA alone to treat resistant infections (US Congress, Office of Technology Assessment, 1995)). It is imperative that clinicians have a high index of suspicion for MRSA so they can promptly initiate the appropriate antibiotic therapy. Failure to act quickly can lead to increased morbidity and mortality for patients. As more virulent strains and increasing resistance occur due to the dynamic nature of this organism, MRSA will remain a growing menace to patients and clinicians. Focused continued education of physicians should improve recognition and treatment, decrease unnecessary antibiotic use, and help reduce the spread of MRSA.

Nevertheless, there is a need for new antimicrobial agents for the treatment of human pathogens that are not susceptible to currently available antibiotics (Wenzel, 2004; Rice, 2003). These development efforts must be coordinated with aggressive infection control efforts and rational use of currently available and emerging antimicrobial agents (Rice, 2003).

REFERENCES

Abbanat D, Macielag M, Bush K. Novel antibacterial agents for the treatment of serious Gram-positive infections. *Expert Opin Invest Drugs* 2003; 12: 379–399.

Adcock PM, Pastor P, Medley F, Patterson JE, Murphy TV. Methicillin resistant *Staphylococcus aureus* in two child care centers. *J Infect Dis* 1998; 178:577-580.

Aeschlimann JR, Rybak MJ. Pharmacodynamic analysis of the activity of quinupristin-dalfopristin against vancomycin resistant Enrerococcus fuecium with differing MBCs via time-kill-curve and postantibiotic effect methods. *Antimicrob Agents Chemothe,:* 1998;42:2188-2192.

Aiello AE, Lowy FD, Wright LN, Larson EL. Methicillin-resistant *Staphylococcus aureus* among US prisoners and military personnel: review and recommendations for future studies. *Lancet Infect Dis* 2006;6:335-341.

Allington DR, Rivey MR. Quinupristin Dalfopristin: A Therapeutic Review. *Clin Therapeut* 2001; 23(1):24-44.

Al-Nammari SS, Bobak P, Venkatesh R. Methicillin resistant *Staphylococcus aureus* versus methicillin sensitive *Staphylococcus aureus* adult haematogenous septic arthritis. *Arch Orthop Trauma Surg* 2007; 127:537-542.

American Thoracic Society, Infectious Diseases Society of America. Guidelines for the management of adults with hospital-acquired, ventilator-associated, and healthcare-associated pneumonia. *Am J Respir Crit Care Med* 2005;171:388-416.

Anon. Four pediatric deaths from community-acquired methicillin-resistant *Staphylococcus aureus* Minnesota and North Dakota. *Morb Mortal Wkly Rep* 1999;48:707-710.

Anstead GM, Owens AD. Recent advances in the treatment of infections due to resistant *Staphylococcus aureus*. *Curr Opin Infect Dis* 2004; 17: 549–555.

Arathoon EG, Hamilton JR, Hench CE, Stevens DA. Efficacy of short courses of oral novobiocin-rifampin in eradicating carrier state of methicillin resistant *Staphylococcus aureus* and in vitro killing studies of clinical isolates. *Antimicrob Agents Chemother* 1990; 34: 1655-1659.

Arbeit RD, Maki D, Tally FP, Campanaro E, Eisenstein BI. The safety and efficacy of daptomycin for the treatment of complicated skin and skin-structure infections. *Clin Infect Dis* 2004; 38: 1673-1681.

Arnold SR, Elias D, Buckingham SC, Thomas ED, Novais E, Arkader A, Howard C. Changing patterns of acute hematogenous osteomyelitis and septic arthritis: emergence of community-associated methicillin resistant *Staphylococcus aureus*. *J Pediatr Orthop.* 2006; 26:703-708.

Attwood RJ, LaPlante KL. Telavancin: a novel lipoglycopeptide antimicrobial agent. *Am J Health Syst Pharm* 2007;64:2335-2348.

Baba T, Takeuchi F, Kuroda M, Yuzawa H, Aoki K, Oguchi A, Nagai Y, Iwama N, Asano K, Naimi T, Kuroda H, Cui L, Yamamoto K, Hiramatsu K. Genome and virulence determinants of high-virulence community acquired MRSA. *Lancet* 2002;359:1819-1827.

Baddour MM, Abuelkheir MM, Fatani AJ. Comparison of *mec*A PCR and phenotypic methods for the detection of MRSA. *Curr Microbiol* 2007a; 55(6): 473-479.

Baddour MM, Abuelkheir MM, Fatani AJ, Bohol M, Alahdal M. Molecular epidemiology of Methicillin Resistant *Staphylococcus aureus* (MRSA) isolates from major hospitals in Riyadh, Saudi Arabia. *Canadian Journal of Microbiology* 2007b; 53 (8): 931-936.

Baddour MM, Abuelkheir MM, Fatani AJ. Trends in antibiotic susceptibility patterns and epidemiology of MRSA isolates from several hospitals in Riyadh, Saudi Arabia. *Annals of Clinical Microbiology and Antimicrobials* 2006; 5: 30.

Barber M. Staphylococcal infection due to penicillin-resistant strains. *Br Med J.* 1947;863-865.

Barbour A, Schmidt S, Rand KH, Derendorf H. Ceftobiprole: a novel cephalosporin with activity against Gram-positive and Gram-negative pathogens, including methicillin-resistant *Staphylococcus aureus* (MRSA). *International Journal of Antimicrobial Agents 2009*, in press.

Begier EM, Frenette K, Barrett NL, Mshar P, Petit S, Boxrud DJ, Watkins-Colwell K, Wheeler S, Cebelinski EA, Glennen A, Nguyen D, Hadler JL; Connecticut Bioterrorism Field Epidemiology Response Team. A high-morbidity outbreak of methicillin resistant *Staphylococcus aureus* among players on a college football team, facilitated by cosmetic body shaving and turf burns. *Clin Infect Dis* 2004;39: 1446-1453.

Bell J. Hand hygiene blamed for neonatal MRSA cases. *Skin Allergy News* 2006;37:6.

Berger-Bachi B, Rohrer S. Factors influencing methicillin resistance in Staphylococci. *Arch Microbiol* 2002; 178:165-171.

Bhalla A, Pultz N, Gries D, Ray AJ, Eckstein EC, Aron DC, Donskey CJ. Acquisition of nosocomial pathogens on hands alter contact with environmental surfaces near hospitalized patients. *Infect Control Hosp Epidemiol* 2004;25:164-167.

Biedenbach DJ, Moet GJ, Jones RN. Occurrence and antimicrobial resistance pattern comparisons among bloodstream infection isolates from the SENTRY Antimicrobial Surveillance Program (1997–2002). *Diagn Microbiol Infect Dis* 2004; 50: 59-69.

Billeter M, Zervos MJ, Chen AY, Dalovisio JR, Kurukularatne C. Dalbavancin: a novel once-weekly lipoglycopeptide antibiotic. *Clin Infect Dis* 2008;46: 577-583.

Bitar CM, Mayhall CG, Lamb VA, Bradshaw TJ, Spadora AC, Dalton HP. Outbreak due to methicillin-resistant *Staphylococcus aureus*: epidemiology and eradication of the resistant strain from the hospital. *Infect Control* 1987; 8: 15-23.

Borg MA, Cookson BD, Rasslan O, Ben Redjeb S, Benbachir M, Rahal K, Bagatzouni DP, Elnasser Z, Daoud Z, Scicluna EA. Correlation between methicillin-resistant *Staphylococcus aureus* prevalence and infection control initiatives within southern and eastern Mediterranean hospitals. *J Hosp Infect* 2009;71(1):36-42.

Boyce JM, Kelliher S, Vallande N. Skin irritation and dryness associated with two hand-hygiene regimens: soap-and-water hand washing versus hand antisepsis with an alcoholic hand gel. *Infect Control Hosp Epidemiol* 2000;21:442-448.

Boyce JM. Methicillin-resistant *Staphylococcus aureus*: detection, epidemiology, and control measures. *Infect Dis Clin North Am* 1989;3:901-913.

Boyle-Vavra S, Daum RS. Community-acquired methicillin-resistant *Staphylococcus aureus*: the role of Panton-Valentine leukocidin. *Lab Invest* 2007;87:3-9.

Bradley SF. *Staphylococcus aureus* pneumonia: emergence of MRSA in the community. *Semin Respir Crit Care Med* 2005;26:643-649.

Bratu S, Eramo A, Kopec R, Coughlin E, Ghitan M, Yost R, Chapnick EK, Landman D, Quale J. Community-associated methicillin-resistant *Staphylococcus aureus* in hospital nursery and maternity units. *Emerg Infec Dis* 2005;11:808-813.

Bryan CS, Wilson RS, Meade P, Sill LG. Topical antibiotic ointments for staphylococcal nasal carriers: survey of current practices and comparison of bacitracin and vancomycin ointments. *Infect Control* 1981; 1: 153-156.

Buckingham SC, McDougal LK, Cathey LD, Comeaux K, Craig AS, Fridkin SK, Tenover FC. Emergence of community-associated methicillin-resistant *Staphylococcus aureus* at a Memphis, Tennessee Children's Hospital. *Pediatr Infect Dis J* 2004; 23: 619-624.

Buescher ES. Community-acquired methicillin-resistant *Staphylococcus aureus* in pediatrics. *Curr Opin Pediatr* 2005; 17:67-70.

Byers DK, Decker CF. The Changing Epidemiology of Methicillin-Resistant *Staphylococcus aureus. Dis Mon* 2008;54:756-762

Campbell KM, Vaugh AF, Russell KL, Smith B, Jimenez DL, Barrozo CP, Minarcik JR, Crum NF, Ryan MA. Risk factors for community-associated methicillin-resistant *Staphylococcus aureus* infections in an outbreak of disease among military trainees in San Diego, California, in 2002. *J Clin Microbiol* 2004;42(9):4050-4053.

Carleton HA, Diep BA, Charlebois ED, Sensabaugh GF, Perdreau-Remington F. Community-adapted methicillin-resistant *Staphylococcus aureus* (MRSA): population dynamics of an expanding community reservoir of MRSA. *J Infect Dis.* 2004;190: 1730-1738.

Caron F, Gold HS, Wennersten CB, , Farris MG, Moellering RC Jr, Eliopoulos GM. Influence of erythromycin resistance, in-oculum growth phase, and incubation time on assessment of the bactericidal activity of RP 59500 (quinupristin-dalfopristin) against vancomycin-resistant Enterococcus faecium. *Antimicrob Agents Chemother* 1997;41:2749-2753.

Casey AL, Worthington T, Caddick JM, Hilton AC, Lambert PA, Elliott TSJ. RAPD for the typing of *Staphylococcus aureus* implicated in nosocomial Infection. *J Hosp Infect* 2007;66: 192-193.

Castaldo ET, Yang EY. Severe sepsis attributable to community associated methicillin-resistant *Staphylococcus aureus*: an emerging fatal problem. *Am Surg* 2007; 73:684-687.

Catherine F. Decker. Pathogenesis of MRSA Infections. *Dis Mon* 2008;54:774-779

Cenizal MJ, Skiest D, Luber S, Bedimo R, Davis P, Fox P, Delaney K, Hardy RD. Prospective randomized trial of empiric therapy with trimethoprim–sulfamethoxazole or doxycycline for outpatient skin and soft tissue infections in an area of high prevalence of methicillin-resistant *Staphylococcus aureus*. *Antimicrob Agents Chemother* 2007; 51:2628-2630.

Centers for Disease Control and Prevention (CDC). Methicillin-resistant *Staphylococcus aureus* infections among competitive sports participants— Colorado, Indiana, Pennsylvania, and Los Angeles county, 2000-2003. *MMWR Morb Mortal Wkly Rep* 2003a;52:793-795.

Centers for Disease Control and Prevention. Outbreaks of community associated methicillin-resistant *Staphylococcus aureus* skin infections — Los Angeles County, California, 2002-2003. MMWR *Morb Mortal Wkly Rep* 2003b;52(5):88.

Centers for Disease Control and Prevention. Community-associated methicillin resistant *Staphylococcus aureus* infections in Pacific Islanders-Hawaii, 2001-2003. *MMWR Morb Mortal Wkly Rep* 2004;53:767-770.

Centers for Disease Control and Prevention. Community-associated MRSA information for clinicians. Available at: http://www.cdc.gov/ncidod/dhqp/ ar_mrsa_ca_clinicians.html. Accessed April 2007.

Centers for Disease Control and Prevention. Four pediatric deaths from community-acquired methicillin-resistant *Staphylococcus aureus* - Minnesota and North Dakota, 1997-1999. *JAMA* 1999;282:1123-1125.

Centers for Disease Control and Prevention. Infectious disease and dermatologic conditions in evacuees and rescue workers after Katrina— Multiple states August–September 2005. *MMWR Morb Mortal Wkly Rep* 2005;54:961-964.

Centers for Disease Control and Prevention. *Staphylococcus aureus* resistant to vancomycin: United States, 2002. *MMWR Morb Mortal Wkly Rep* 2002;51: 565-567.

Centers for Disease Control and Prevention: Methicillin-resistant *Staphylococcus aureus* skin or soft tissue infections in a state prison: Mississippi, 2000. *MMWR Morb Mortal Wkly Rep* 2001;50:919-922.

Centers for Disease Control. Methicillin resistant *Staphylococcus aureus* skin infections among tattoo recipients—Ohio, Kentucky and Vermont, 2004-2005. *MMWR Morb Mortal Wkly Rep* 2006;55:677-679.

Centers for Disease Control. Methicillin-resistant *Staphylococcus aureus* skin or soft tissue infections in a state prison: Mississippi, 2000. *MMWR Morb Mortal Wkly Rep* 2001;50:919-922.

Cercenado E, Cercenado S, Gomez JA, Bouza E. In vitro activity of tigecycline (GAR-936), a novel glycylcycline, against vancomycin-resistant enterococci and staphylococci with diminished susceptibility to glycopeptides. *J Antimicrob Chemother* 2003;52:138–139.

Chamberland S, Blais J, Hoang M, Park C, Chan C, Mathias K, Hakem S, Dupree K, Liu E, Nguyen T, Dudley MN. In vitro activities of RWJ-54428 (MC-02,479) against multiresistant gram-positive bacteria. *Antimicrob Agents Chemother* 2001; 45: 1422– 1430.

Chambers HF. In vitro and in vivo antistaphylococcal activities of L-695,256, a carbapenem with high affinity for the penicillin-binding protein PBP 2a. *Antimicrob Agents Chemother* 1995; 39: 462–466.

Chambers HF. Methicillin resistance in Staphylococci: molecular and biochemical basis and clinical implications. *Clin Microbiol Rev* 1997;10:781-791.

Chambers HF. Solving staphylococcal resistance to betalactams. *Trends Microbiol* 2003; 11: 145–148.

Chambers, HF. The changing epidemiology of *Staphylococcus aureus*? *Emerg Infect Dis* 2001; 7: 178-182.

Chang FY, Peacock JE, Jr., Musher DM, Triplett P, MacDonald BB, Mylotte JM, O'Donnell A, Wagener MM, Yu VL. *Staphylococcus aureus* bacteremia: recurrence and the impact of antibiotic treatment in a prospective multicenter study. *Medicine (Baltimore)* 2003; 82: 333-339.

Chang FY, Singh N, Gayowski T, Drenning SD, Wagener MM, Marino IR. *Staphylococcus aureus* nasal colonization and association with infections in liver transplant recipients. *Transplantation* 1998;65:1169-1172.

Charlebois ED, Bangsberg DR, Moss NJ, Moore MR, Moss AR, Chambers HF, Perdreau☐Remington F. Population-based community prevalence of methicillin-resistant *Staphylococcus aureus* in the urban poor of San Francisco. Clin Infect Dis 2002;34:425-433.

Charlebois ED, Perdreau-Reminton F, Kreiswirth B, Bangsberg DR, Ciccarone D, Diep B, Valerie L Ng, Chansky K, Edlin B, Chambers HF. Origins of community strains of methicillin-resistant *Staphylococcus aureus*. *Clin Infect Dis* 2004;39:47-54.

Charles PG, Ward PB, Johnson PD, Howden BP, Grayson ML. Clinical features associated with bacteremia due to heterogeneous vancomycin-intermediate Staphylococcus aureus. *Clin Infect Dis* 2004; 38: 448-451.

Chaves F, Garcia-Martinez J, de Miguel S, Sanz F, Otero JR. Epidemiology and clonality of methicillin-resistant and methicillin-susceptible *Staphylococcus aureus* causing bacteremia in a tertiary-care hospital in Spain. *Infect Control Hosp Epidemiol* 2005; 26:150-156.

Chavez TT, Decker CF. Health Care-Associated MRSA Versus Community-Associated MRSA. *Dis Mon* 2008;54:763-768.

Cheeseman KE, Williams GJ, Maillard J-Y, Denyer, SP, Mahenthiralingam E, Typing of *Staphylococcus aureus* clinical isolates using random amplification of polymorphic DNA method and comparison with antibiotic susceptibility typing. *J Hosp Infect* 2007;67(4):388-390.

Chongtrakool P, Ito T, Ma XX, Kondo Y, Trakulsomboon S, Tiensasitorn C, Jamklang M, Chavalit T, Song JH, Hiramatsu K. Staphylococcal cassette chromosome *mec* (*SCCmec*) typing of methicillin-resistant *Staphylococcus aureus* strains isolated in 11 Asian countries: a proposal for a new nomenclature for *SCCmec* elements. Antimicrob. *Agents Chemother* 2006; 50: 1001-1012.

Cimolai N. MRSA and the environment: implications for comprehensive control measures. *Eur J Clin Microbiol Infect Dis* 2008;27(7):481-493.

Clinical and Laboratory Standards Institute. Performance standards for antimicrobial susceptibility testing: 16th informational supplement. Wayne, PA: Clinical and Laboratory Standards Institute; 2006. M100-S16

CLSI Performance standards for antimicrobial susceptibility testing: seventeenth informational supplement. M100–S17. Wayne, PA: *Clinical and Laboratory Standards Institute,* 2007;52.

Cohen PR. Cutaneous community-acquired methicillin-resistant *Staphylococcus aureus* infection in participants of athletic activities. *South Med J* 2005; 98:596-602.

Cook HA, Furuya EY, Larson E, Vasquez G, Lowy FD. Heterosexual transmission of community-associated methicillin-resistant *Staphylococcus aureus. Clin Infect Dis* 2007; 44:410-413.

Cosgrove SE, Sakoulas G, Perencevich EN, Schwaber MJ, Karchmer AW, Carmeli Y. Comparison of mortality associated with methicillin resistant and methicillin-susceptible *Staphylococcus aureus* bacteremia: a meta-analysis. *Clin Infect Dis* 2003; 36: 53-59.

Crawford DH. *Deadly companions: How microbes shaped our history.* Oxford: Oxford University Press; 2008.

Crowcroft NS, Catchpole M. Mortality from methicillin resistant *Staphylococcus aureus* in England and Wales: analysis of death certificates. *Br Med J* 2002;325:1390-1391.

Cruciani M, Gatti G, Lazzarini L, Furlan G, Broccali G, Malena M, Franchini C, Concia E. Penetration of vancomycin into human lung tissue. *J Antimicrob Chemother* 1996;38:865-869.

Cui L, Murakami H, Kuwahara-Arai K, Hanaki H, Hiramatsu K. Contribution of a thickened cell wall and its gultamine nonamidated component to the vancomycin resistance expressed by *Staphylococcus aureus* Mu50. *Antimicrob Agents Chemother* 2000; 44: 2276-2285.

Cui L, Tominaga E, Neoh HM, Hiramatsu K. Correlation between reduced daptomycin susceptibility and vancomycin resistance in vancomycin-intermediate *Staphylococcus aureus*. *Antimicrob Agents Chemother 2006;* 50: 1079-1082.

Dancer SJ. Keeping watch over the Staphylococcus. *J Hosp Infect* 2008; 70: 297.

Darouiche R, Wright C, Hamill R, Koza M, Lewis D, Markowski J. Eradication of colonization by methicillin-resistant *Staphylococcus aureus* by using oral minocycline–rifampin and topical mupirocin. *Antimicrob Agents Chemother* 1991; 35: 1612-1615.

Daum RS, Ito T, Hiramatsu K, Hussain F, Mongkolrattanothai K, Jamklang M, Boyle-Vavra S. A novel methicillin-resistance cassette in community-acquired methicillin-resistant *Staphylococcus aureus* isolates of diverse genetic backgrounds. J Infect Dis 2002; 186:1344-1347.

Daum RS. Community-acquired methicillin-resistant *Staphylococcus aureus* infections. *Pediatr Infect Dis J* 1998; 17:745-746.

Daum RS. Skin and soft-tissue infections caused by methicillin-resistant *Staphylococcus aureus*. *N Engl J Med* 2007;357:280-290.

Daver NG, Shelburne SA, Atmar RL, Giordano TP, Stager CE, Reitman CA, White AC Jr. Oral step-down therapy is comparable to intravenous therapy for *Staphylococcus aureus* osteomyelitis. *Journal of Infection* 2007; 54(6):539-544.

David MZ, Glikman D, Crawford SE, Peng J, King KJ, Hostetler MA, Boyle-Vavra S, Daum RS. What Is community-associated methicillin-resistant *Staphylococcus aureus*? *J Infect Dis* 2008; 197: 1235-1243.

Davis KA, Stewart JJ, Crouch HK, Florez CE, Hospenthal DR. Methicillin-resistant *Staphylococcus aureus* (MRSA) nares colonization at hospital admission and its effect on subsequent MRSA infection. *Clin Infect Dis* 2004;39 (6):776-782.

Decker BS, Babel CF. Microbiology and Laboratory Diagnosis of MRSA. Dis Mon 2008;54:769-773

Denis O, Nonhoff C, Byl B, Knoop C, Bobin-Dubreux S, Struelens MJ. Emergence of vancomycin-intermediate *Staphylococcus aureus* in a Belgian hospital: microbiological and clinical features. *J Antimicrob Chemother* 2002; 50: 383-391.

Deresinski S. Counterpoint: Vancomycin and *Staphylococcus aureus* an antibiotic enters obsolescence. *Clin Infect Dis* 2007a; 44: 1543-1548.

Deresinski S. Principles of antibiotic therapy in severe infections: optimizing the therapeutic approach by use of laboratory and clinical data. *Clin Infect Dis* 2007b; 45:177-183.

Deshpande L, Rhomberg PR, Fritsche TR, Sader HS, Jones RN. Bactericidal activity of BAL9141, a novel parenteral cephalosporin against contemporary Gram-positive and Gram-negative isolates. *Diagn Microbiol Infect Dis* 2004;50: 73–75.

Deurenberg RH, Vink C, Kalenic S, Friedrich AW, Bruggeman CA, Stobberingh EE. The molecular evolution of methicillin resistant *Staphylococcus aureus. Clin Microbiol Infect* 2007;13 (3):222-235.

Diederen BM, Kluytmans JA. The emergence of infections with community associated methicillin resistant *Staphylococcus aureus. J Infect* 2006;52:157-168.

Diep BA, Carleton HA, Chang RF, Friedrich AW, Bruggeman CA, Stobberingh EE. Role of 34 virulence genes in the evolution of hospital- and community-associated strains of methicillin-resistant *Staphylococcus aureus. J Infect Dis 2006a;*193:1495-1503.

Diep BA, Chambers HF, Graber CJ, Szumowski JD, Miller LG, Han LL, Chen JH, Lin F, Lin J, Phan TH, Carleton HA, McDougal LK, Tenover FC, Cohen DE, Mayer KH, Sensabaugh GF, Perdreau-Remington F. Emergence of multidrug-resistant, community-associated, methicillin-resistant *Staphylococcus aureus* clone USA200 in men who have sex with men. *Ann Intern Med* 2008;148:249-257.

Diep BA, Gill SR, Chang RF, Phan TH, Chen JH, Davidson MG, Lin F, Lin J, Carleton HA, Mongodin EF, SensabaughGF, Perdreau-Remington F. Complete genome sequence of USA300, an epidemic clone of community-acquired methicillin-resistant *Staphylococcus aureus. Lancet* 2006b;367:731-739.

Diep BA, Stone GG, Basuino L, Graber CJ, Miller A, des Etages SA, Jones A, Palazzolo-Ballance AM, Perdreau-Remington F, Sensabaugh GF, DeLeo FR, Chambers HF. The arginine catabolic mobile element and staphylococcal chromosomal cassette mec linkage: convergence of virulence and resistance in the USA300clone of methicillin-resistant *Staphylococcus aureus*. *J Infect Dis* 2008;97(11):1523-1530.

Dietze B, Rath A, Wendt C, Martiny H. Survival of MRSA on sterile goods packaging. J Hosp Infect 2001;49: 255-261.

Dombrowski JC, Winston LG. Clinical failures of appropriately-treated methicillin-resistant *Staphylococcus aureus* infections. *Journal of Infection* 2008; 57: 110-115.

Drekonja DM, Traynor LM, DeCarolis DD, Crossley KB, Johnson JR. Treatment of non–life-threatening methicillin-resistant *Staphylococcus aureus* infections with alternative antimicrobial agents: a 2-year retrospective review. *Diagnostic Microbiology and Infectious Disease* 2009; 63(2):201-207.

Duckworth G, Cookson B, Humphreys H, Heathcock R. Working party report. Revised guidelines for the control of methicillin-resistant *Staphylococcus aureus* infection in hospitals. *J Hosp Infect* 1998; 39: 253-290.

Duckworth G. Improving surveillance of MRSA bacteraemia. *Br Med J* 2005;331:976-977.

Eady EA, Cove JH. Staphylococcal resistance revisited: community-acquired methicillin resistant *Staphylococcus aureus*-an emerging problem for the management of skin and soft tissue infections. *Curr Opin Infect Dis* 2003;16:103-124.

ElKamel A, Baddour MM. Gatifloxacin-biodegradable implant for treatment of experimental osteomyelitis. In vitro and in vivo evaluation. *Drug Delivery* 2007; 14 (6): 349-356.

Ellis MW, Hospenthal DR, Dooley DP, Gray PJ, Murray CK. Natural history of community-acquired methicillin-resistant *Staphylococcus aureus* colonization and infection in soldiers. *Clin Infect Dis* 2004; 39: 971-979.

Enoch DA, Karas JA, Aliyu SH. Oral antimicrobial options for the treatment of skin and soft-tissue infections caused by methicillin-resistant *Staphylococcus aureus* (MRSA) in the UK. *Int. J. Antimicrob. Agents* (2008), doi:10.1016/j.ijantimicag.2008.10.014

Enright MC, Spratt BG. Multilocus sequence typing. *Trends in Microbiology* 1999; 7: 482-487.

Esposito AL, Gleckman RA. Vancomycin: a second look. *J Am Med Assoc* 1977; 238:1756-1757.

Etienne J. Panton-Valentine leukocidin: a marker of severity for *Staphylococcus aureus* infection? *Clin Infect Dis* 2005; 41: 591-593.

Euzéby JP. Definitions and abbreviatons. J.P. Euzéby: *List of Bacteria Names with Standing in Nomenclature.* 2004 http://www.bacterio.cict.fr2004.

Falagas ME, Giannopoulou KP, Ntziora F, Vardakas KZ. Daptomycin for endocarditis and/or bacteraemia: a systematic review of the experimental and clinical evidence. *J Antimicrob Chemother* 2007;60:7-19.

Farley JE, Ross T, Stamper P, Baucom S, Larson E, Carroll KC. Prevalence, risk factors, and molecular epidemiology of methicillin-resistant *Staphylococcus aureus* among newly arrested men in Baltimore, Maryland. *Am J Infect Control* 2008;36:644-650.

Flynn N, Cohen SH. The continuing saga of MRSA. *J Infect Dis* 2008;197:1217-1219.

Fowler VG Jr, Kong LK, Corey GR, Gottlieb GS, McClelland RS, Sexton DJ, Gesty-Palmer D, Harrell LJ. Recurrent *Staphylococcus aureus* bacteremia: pulsed-field gel electrophoresis findings in 29 patients. *J Infect Dis* 1999;179:1157-1161.

Fowler VG Jr, Sexton DJ. Complications of *Staphylococcus aureus* bacteremia. In: Rose BD, editor. *UpToDate.* (Database online and on CD-ROM). Wellesley, Mass: UpToDate; 2001.

Fowler VG Jr., Boucher HW, Corey GR, Abrutyn E, Karchmer AW, Rupp ME, Levine DP, Chambers HF, Tally FP, Vigliani GA, Cabell CH, Link AS, DeMeyer I, Filler SG, Zervos M, Cook P, Parsonnet J, Bernstein JM, Price CS, Forrest GN, Fatkenheuer G, Gareca M, Rehm SJ, Brodt HR, Tice A, Cosgrove SE. Daptomycin versus standard therapy for bacteremia and endocarditis caused by *Staphylococcus aureus. N Engl J Med* 2006; 355: 653-665.

Fraise AP. Guidelines for the control of methicillin resistant *Staphylococcus aureus. J Antimicrob Chemother* 1998; 42: 287-289.

Francis JS, Doherty MC, Lopatin U, Johnston CP, Sinha G, Ross T, Cai M, Hansel NN, Perl T, Ticehurst JR, Carroll K, Thomas DL, Nuermberger E, Bartlett JG. Severe community-onset pneumonia in healthy adults caused by methicillin-resistant *Staphylococcus aureus* carrying the Panton-Valentine leukocidin genes. *Clin Infect Dis* 2005;40:100-107.

Fraser C, Riley S, Anderson RM, Ferguson NM. Factors that make an infectious disease outbreak controllable. *Proc Natl Acad Sci U S A* 2004; 101:6146-6151.

Frenay HM, Bunschoten AE, Schouls LM, van Leeuwen WJ, Vandenbroucke-Grauls CM, Verhoef J, Mooi FR. Molecular typing of methicillin resistant *Staphylococcus aureus* on the basis of protein A gene polymorphism. *Eur J Clin Microbiol Infect Dis* 1996; 15: 60-64.

Fridkin SK, Hageman J, McDougal LK , Mohammed J, Jarvis WR, Perl TM, Tenover FC; Vancomycin-Intermediate *Staphylococcus aureus* Epidemiology Study Group. Epidemiological and microbiological characterization of infections caused by *Staphylococcus aureus* with reduced susceptibility to vancomycin, United States, 1997–2001. *Clin Infect Dis* 2003; 36: 429-439.

Fridkin SK, Hageman JC, Morrison M, Sanza LT, Como-Sabetti K, Jernigan JA, Harriman K, Harrison LH, Lynfield R, Farley MM; Active Bacterial Core Surveillance Program of the Emerging Infections Program Network. Methicillin-resistant *Staphylococcus aureus* disease in three communities. *N Engl J Med* 2005;352:1436-1444.

Fritsche TR, Sader HS, Jones RN. Antimicrobial activity of ceftobiprole, a novel anti-methicillin-resistant *Staphylococcus aureus* cephalosporin, tested against contemporary pathogens: results from the SENTRY Antimicrobial Surveillance Program (2005–2006). *Diagn Microbiol Infect Dis* 2008;61:86–95.

Fuchs PC, Barry AL, Brown SD. Evaluation of daptomycin susceptibility testing by E-test and the effect of different batches of media. *J Antimicrob Chemother* 2001;48:557-561.

Gales AC, Sader HS, Andrade SS, Lutz L, Machado A, Barth AL. Emergence of linezolid-resistant *Staphylococcus aureus* during treatment of pulmonary infection in a patient with cystic fibrosis. *Int J Antimicrob Agents* 2006; 27:300-302.

Gang RK, Sanyal SC, Bang RL, Mokaddas E, Lari AR. Staphylococcal septicaemia in burns. *Burns* 2000;26:359-366.

Garazzino S, Aprato A, Baietto L, D'Avolio A, Maiello A, De Rosa FG, Aloj D, Siccardi M, Biasibetti A, Massè A, Di Perri G. Glycopeptide bone penetration in patients with septic pseudoarthrosis of the tibia. *Clin Pharmacokinet.* 2008;47(12):793-805.

Garnier F, Tristan A, Francois B, Etienne J, Delage-Corre M, Martin C, Liassine N, Wannet W, Denis F, Ploy MC. Pneumonia and new methicillin-resistant *Staphylococcus aureus* clone. *Emerg Infect Dis* 2006;12:498-500.

Garrity GM, Holt JG. 2001. The road map to the manual. In: Boone, R.D., Castenholz, R.W., Garrity, G.M. (Eds.), *Bergey's Manual of Systematic Bacteriology,* 2nd ed. Springer-Verlag, New York, NY, pp. 119-166.

Gentry CA, Rodvold KA, Novak RM, Hershow RC, Naderer OJ. Retrospective evaluation of therapies for *Staphylococcus aureus* endocarditis. *Pharmacotherapy* 1997; 17: 990-997.

Giammarinaro P, Leroy S, Chacornac JP, Delmas J, Talon R. Development of a new oligonucleotide array to identify staphylococcal strains at species level. *J Clin Microbiol* 2005; 43 (8): 3673-3680.

Gilbert DN, Mollering RC, Eliopoulos GM, Sande MA, editors. *The Sanford guide to antimicrobial therapy.* Sperryville, VA: Antimicrobial Therapy, Inc.; 2007.

Gilbert M, MacDonald J, Gregson D, Siushansian J, Zhang K, Elsayed S, Laupland K, Louie T, Hope K, Mulvey M, Gillespie J, Nielsen D, Wheeler V, Louie M, Honish A, Keays G, Conly J. Outbreak in Alberta of community acquired methicllin-resistant *Staphylococcus aureus* in people with a history of drug abuse, homelessness or incarceration. *CMAJ* 2006;175:149-154.

Gillett Y, Issartel B, Vanhems P, Fournet JC, Lina G, Bes M, Vandenesch F, Piémont Y, Brousse N, Floret D, Etienne J. Association between *Staphylococcus aureus* strains carrying gene for Panton-Valentine leukocidin and highly lethal necrotizing pneumonia in young immunocompetent patients. *Lancet* 2002;359:753-759.

Gonzales RD, Schreckenberger PC, Graham MB, Kelkar S, DenBesten K, Quinn JP. Infections due to vancomycin-resistant Enterococcus faecium resistant to linezolid. *Lancet* 2001; 357:1179.

Gonzalez C, Rubio M, Romero-Vivas J, Gonzalez M, Picazo JJ. Bacteremic pneumonia due to *Staphylococcus aureus*: a comparison of disease caused by methicillin-resistant and methicillin-susceptible organisms. *Clin Infect Dis* 1999; 29: 1171–1177.

Gordin FM, Schultz ME, Huber RA, Gill JA. Reduction in nosocomial transmission of drug-resistant bacteria after introduction of an alcohol-based handrub. *Infect Control Hosp Epidemiol* 2005;26:650-653.

Gorwitz RJ, Jemigan DB, Powers JH. Strategies for clinical management of MRSA in the community: summary of an experts' meeting convened by the Centers for Disease Control and Prevention. March 2006. Available at: http://www.cdc.gov/ncidod/dhqp/ pdf/ar/CAMRSA_ExpMtgStrategies.pdf. Accessed May 20, 2008.

Gorwitz RJ, Jernigan DB, Powers JH. Strategies for clinical management of MRSA in the community: summary of an experts' meeting convened by the Centers for Disease Control and Prevention, 2006. Available at: http://www.cdc.gov/ncidod/dhqp/ar_mrsa_ca.html. Accessed May 15, 2008.

Gorwitz RJ. The role of ancillary antimicrobial therapy for treatment of uncomplicated skin infections in the era of community-associated methicillin-resistant Staphylococcus aureus. *Clin Infect Dis* 2007;44:785-787.

Gould I. Clinical relevance of increasing glycopeptide MICs against Staphylococcus aureus. *Int J Antimicrob Agents* 2008; 31:1-9.

Gould IM. Costs of hospital-acquired methicillin-resistant *Staphylococcus aureus* (MRSA) and its control. *Int J Antimicrob Agents* 2006;28:379-384.

Gould IM. MRSA bacteraemia. *Int J Antimicrob Agents* 2007b; 30 Suppl 1: S66-S70.

Gould IM. The problem with glycopeptides. *Int J Antimicrob Agents* 2007a; 30: 1-3.

Gradon JD, Wu EH, Lutwick LI. Aerosolized vancomycin therapy facilitating nursing home placement. *Ann Pharmacother* 1992; 26: 209-210.

Graffunder EM, Venezia RA. Risk factors associated with noscomial methicillin resistant *Staphylococcus aureus* (MRSA) infection including previous use of antimicrobials. *J Antimicrob Chemother* 2002;49:999-1005.

Groom AV, Wolsey DH, Naimi TS, Smith K, Johnson S, Boxrud D, Moore KA, Cheek JE. Community-associated methcillin resistant *Staphylococcus aureus* in a rural American Indian community. *J Am Med Assoc* 2001;286:1201-1205.

Grundmann H, Aires-de-Sousa M, Boyce J, Tiemersma E. Emergence and resurgence of methicillin-resistant *Staphylococcus aureus* as a public-health threat. *Lancet* 2006; 368(9538):874-885.

Gur D, Unal S. Resistance to antimicrobial agents in Mediterranean countries. *Int J Antimicrob Agents* 2001; 17:21-26.

Hahn RC, Macedo AM, Fontes CJF, Batista RD, Santos NL, Hamdan S. Randomly amplified polymorphic DNA as a valuable tool for epidemiological studies of Paracoccidioides brasiliensis. *J Clin Microbiol* 2003;41:2849-2854.

Hails J, Kwaku F, Wilson AP, Bellingan G, Singer M. Large variation in MRSA policies, procedures and prevalence in English intensive care units: a questionnaire analysis. *Intensive Care Med* 2003;29:481-483.

Harbarth S, Dharan S, Liassine N, Herrault P, Auckenthaler R, Pittet D. Randomized, placebo controlled, double-blind trial to evaluate the efficacy of mupirocin for eradicating carriage of methicillin-resistant Staphylococcus aureus. *Antimicrob Agents Chemother* 1999; 43: 1412-1416.

Hayden MK, Rezai K, Hayes RA, Lolans K, Quinn JP, Weinstein RA. Development of Daptomycin resistance in vivo in methicillin-resistant Staphylococcus aureus. *J Clin Microbiol.* 2005;43: 5285-5287.

Health Protection Agency, 2005. *Staphylococcus aureus bacteraemia laboratory reports and methicillin susceptibility* (voluntary reporting scheme): England and Wales, 1990–2003. http://www.hpa.org.uk/ infections/ topics az/staphylo/lab data staphyl.htm. [Accessed May 2007].

Healy M, Huong J, Bittner T, Lising M, Frye S, Raza S, Schrock R, Manry J, Renwick A, Nieto R, Woods C, Versalovic J, Lupski JR. Microbial DNA typing by automated repetitive-sequence-based PCR. *J Clin Microbiol* 2005; 43:199-207.

Hebeisen P, Heinze-Krauss I, Angehrn P, Hohl P, Page MG, Then RL. In vitro and in vivo properties of Ro 63- 9141, a novel broad-spectrum cephalosporin with activity against methicillin-resistant staphylococci. *Antimicrob Agents Chemother* 2001; 45: 825–836.

Herold BC, Immergluck LC, Maranan MC, Lauderdale DS, Gaskin RE, Boyle-Vavra S, Leitch CD, Daum RS. Community-acquired methicillin-resistant *Staphylococcus aureus* in children with no identified predisposing risk. *JAMA* 1998; 279:593-598.

Herrera MO, Gallegos AG, Schacht FC, Fernandez LP, Jimenez RC. RAPD-PCR characterization of Pseudomonas aeruginosa strains obtained from cystic fibrosis patients. *Salud Publica Mex* 2004;46:149-157.

Hill RLR, Duckworth GJ, Casewell NW. Elimination of nasal carriage of methicillin resistant *Staphylococcus aureus* with mupirocin during a hospital outbreak. *J Antimicrob Chemother* 1998; 22: 377-384.

Hiramatsu K, Aritaka N, Hanaki H, Kawasaki S, Hosoda Y, Hori S, Fukuchi Y, Kobayashi I. Dissemination in Japanese hospitals of strains of *Staphylococcus aureus* heterogeneously resistant to vancomycin. *Lancet* 1997;350:1670-1673.

Hiramatsu K, Hanaki H, Ino T, Yabuta K, Oguri T, Tenover FC. Methicillin-resistant *Staphylococcus aureus* clinical strain with reduced vancomycin susceptibility. *J Antimicrob Chemother* 1997; 40: 135-136.

Hiramatsu K. Vancomycin-resistant Staphylococcus aureus: a new model of antibiotic resistance. *Lancet Infect Dis* 2001; 1: 147-155

Hisata K, Kuwahara-Arai K, Yamanoto M, Ito T, Nakatomi Y, Cui L, Baba T, Terasawa M, Sotozono C, Kinoshita S, Yamashiro Y, Hiramatsu K. Dissemination of methicillin-resistant staphylococci among healthy Japanese children. *J Clin Microbiol* 2005; 43:3364-3372.

Hoellman DB, Pankuch GA, Jacobs MR, AppelbaumPC. Antipneumococcal activities of GAR-936 (a new glycylcycline) compared to those of nine other agents against penicillin-susceptible and -resistant pneumococci. *Antimicrob Agents Chemothe*r 2000;44:1085-1088.

Hood J, Edwards GFS, Cosgrove B, Curran E, Morrison D, Gemmell CG. Vancomycin-intermediate *Staphylococcus aureus* at a Scottish hospital. *J Infect* 2000;40:A11.

Howden BP, Ward PB, Charles PG Korman TM, Fuller A, du Cros P, Grabsch EA, Roberts SA, Robson J, Read K, Bak N, Hurley J, Johnson PD, Morris AJ, Mayall BC, Grayson ML. Treatment outcomes for serious infections caused by methicillin-resistant *Staphylococcus aureus* with reduced vancomycin susceptibility. *Clin Infect Dis* 2004; 38: 521-528.

Howe RA, Wootton M, Noel AR, Bowker KE, Walsh TR, MacGowan AP. Activity of AZD2563, a novel oxazolidinone, against *Staphylococcus aureus* strains with reduced susceptibility to vancomycin or linezolid. *Antimicrob Agents Chemother* 2003; 47: 3651-3652.

Huang R, Mehta S, Weed D, Price CS. Methicillin resistant *Staphylococcus aureus* survival on hospital fomites. *Infect Control Hosp Epidemiol* 2006; 27: 1267-1269.

Huang SS, Platt R. Risk of methicillin-resistant *Staphylococcus aureus* infection after previous infection or colonization. *Clin Infect Dis* 2003;36:281-285.

Huang YH, Tseng SP, Hu JM, Tsai JC, Hsueh PR, Teng LJ. Clonal spread of SCCmec type IV methicillin-resistant *Staphylococcus aureus* between community and hospital. *Clin Microbiol Infect* 2007;13:717-724.

Hueletsky A, Giroux R, Rossbach V, et al. New real-time PCR assay for rapid detection of methicillin resistant *Staphylococcus aureus* directly from specimens containing a mixture of staphylococci. *J Clin Microbiol* 2004;42:1835-1841.

Ibrahim EH, Sherman G, Ward S, Fraser VJ, Kollef MH. The influence of inadequate antimicrobial treatment of bloodstream infections on patient outcomes in the ICU setting. *Chest* 2000;118:9-11.

Iizawa Y, Nagai J, Ishikawa T, Hashiguchi S, Nakao M, Miyake A, Okonogi K. In vitro antimicrobial activity of T-91825, a novel anti-MRSA cephalosporin, and in vivo anti-MRSA activity of its prodrug, TAK-599. *J Infect Chemother* 2004; 10: 146–156.

Infectious Disease Society of America (IDSA). Bad Bugs, No Drugs. *As Antibiotic Discovery Stagnates. A Public Health Crisis Brews.* Alexandria, Va: IDSA; 2004.

Ito T, Katayama Y, Asada K, Mori N, Tsutsumimoto K, Tiensasitorn C, Hiramatsu K. Structural comparison of three types of staphylococcal cassette chromosome mec integrated in the chromosome in methicillin-resistant Staphylococcus aureus. *Antimicrob Agents Chemother* 2001;45: 1323-1336.

Ito T, Ma XX, Takeuchi F, Okuma K, Yuzawa H, Hiramatsu K. Novel type V staphylococcal cassette chromosome mec driven by a novel cassette chromosome recombinase, ccrC. *Antimicrob Agents Chemother* 2004; 48 :2637-2651.

Ito T, Okuma K, Ma XX, Yuzawa H, Hiramatsu K. Insights on antibiotic resistance of *Staphylococcus aureus* from its whole genome: genomic island SCC. *Drug Resist Updat* 2003; 6:41-52.

Iyer S, Jones DH. Community-acquired methicillin-resistant *Staphylococcus aureus* skin infection: a retrospective analysis of clinical presentation and treatment of a local outbreak. *J Am Acad Dermatol* 2004; 50:854-858.

Jansen WT, Beitsma MM, Koeman CJ, van Wamel WJ, Verhoef J, Fluit AC. Novel mobile variants of staphylococcal cassette chromosome mec in Staphylococcus aureus. Antimicrob. *Agents Chemother* 2006: 50: 2072-2078.

Jauregui LE, Babazadeh S, Seltzer E, Goldberg L, Krievins D, Frederick M, Krause D, Satilovs I, Endzinas Z, Breaux J, O'Riordan W. Randomized, double-blind comparison of once-weekly dalbavancin versus twice-daily linezolid therapy for the treatment of complicated skin and skin structure infections. *Clin Infect Dis* 2005;41:1407-1415.

Jeffres MN, Isakow W, Doherty JA, Micek ST, Kollef MH. A retrospective study of possible renal toxicity in patients with healthcare-associated meticillin resistant *Staphylococcus aureus* pneumonia treated with vancomycin. *Clin Ther* 2007;29:1107-1115.

Jevons M. "Celbenin"-resistant staphylococci. *Br Med J.* 1961:124-125.

Johnson AP, Aucken HM, Cavendish S, et al. Dominance of EMRSA-15 and -16 among MRSA causing nosocomial bacteraemia in the UK: analysis of isolates from the European Antimicrobial Resistance Surveillance System (EARSS). *J Antimicrob Chemother* 2001;48:143-144.

Johnson AP, Pearson A, Duckworth G. Surveillance and epidemiology of MRSA bacteraemia in the UK. *J Antimicrob Chemother* 2005;56:455–462.

Jones RN, Della-Latta P, Lee LV, Biedenbach DJ. Linezolid resistant Enterococcus faecium isolated from a patient without prior exposure to an oxazolidinone: report from the SENTRY Antimicrobial Surveillance Program. *Diagn Microbiol Infect Dis* 2002; 42:

Jones RN, Deshpande LM, Mutnick AH, Biedenbach DJ. In vitro evaluation of BAL9141, a novel parenteral cephalosporin active against oxacillin-resistant staphylococci. *J Antimicrob Chemother* 2002;50:915–932.

Kaatz GW, Seo SM, Dorman NJ, Lerner SA. Emergence of teicoplanin resistance during therapy of *Staphylococcus aureus* endocarditis. *J Infect Dis* 1990; 162: 103-108.

Kahl BC, Mellmann A, Deiwick S, Peters G, Harmsen D. Variation of the polymorphic region X of the protein A gene during persistent airway infection of cystic fibrosis patients reflects two independent mechanisms of genetic change in Staphylococcus aureus. *J Clin Microbiol* 2005; 43: 502-505.

Kainer MA, Devasia RA, Jones TF, Simmons BP, Melton K, Chow S, Broyles J, Moore KL, Craig AS, Schaffner W. Response to emerging infection leading to outbreak of linezolid-resistant enterococci. *Emerg Infect Dis* 2007; 13:1024-1030.

Kalteis T, Beckmann J, Schröder HJ, Handel M, Grifka J, Lehn N, Lerch K. Acta Orthop. *Moxifloxacin superior to vancomycin for treatment of bone infections--a study in rats.* 2006;77(2):315-319.

Kaneko J, Kamio Y. Bacterial two-component and hetero-heptameric poreforming cytolytic toxins: structures, pore-forming mechanism, and organization of the genes. *Biosci Biotechnol Biochem* 2004; 68: 981-1003.

Karchmer AW. Nosocomial bloodstream infections: organisms, risk factors and implications. *Clin Infect Dis* 2000;31:S13-43 (suppl 4).

Katayama Y, Ito T, Hiramatsu K. Genetic organization of the chromosome region surrounding mecA in clinical staphylococcal strains: role of IS431-mediated mecI deletion in expression of resistance in mecA-carrying, low-level methicillin-resistant Staphylococcus haemolyticus. *Antimicrob Agents Chemother* 2001;45: 1955-1963.

Kauffman CA, Terpenning MS, He X, Zarins LT, Ramsey MA, Jorgensen KA, Sottile WS, Bradley SF. Attempts to eradicate methicillin-resistant *Staphylococcus aureus* from a long-term-care facility with the use of mupirocin ointment. *Am J Med* 1993; 94: 371-378.

Kazakova SV, Hageman JC, Matava ME, Srinivasan A, Phelan L, Garfinkel B, Boo T, McAllister S, Anderson J, Jensen B, Dodson D, Lonsway D, McDougal LK, Arduino M, Fraser VJ, Killgore G, Tenover FC, Cody S, Jernigan DB. A clone of methicillin-resistant *Staphylococcus aureus* among professional football players. *N Engl J Med* 2005;352:468-475.

Keshtgar MR, Khalili A, Coen PG, Carder C, Macrae B, Jeanes A, Folan P, Baker D, Wren M, Wilson AP. Impact of rapid molecular screening for methicillin-resistant *Staphylococcus aureus* in surgical wards. *Br J Surg* 2008;95:381-386.

Khandavilli S, Wilson P, Cookson B, Cepeda J, Bellingan G, Brown J. Utility of spa typing for investigating the local epidemiology of MRSA on a UK intensive care ward. *J Hosp Infect* 2009;71(1):29-35.

Kim J, Jeong JH, Cha HY, Jin JS, Lee JC, Lee YC, Seol SY, Cho DT. Detection of diverse SCCmec variants in methicillin-resistant *Staphylococcus aureus* and comparison of SCCmec typing methods. *Clin Microbiol Infect* 2007; 13: 1128-1130.

King MD, Humphrey BJ, Wang YF, Kourbatova EV, Ray SM, Blumberg HM. Emergence of community-acquired methicillin-resistant *Staphylococcus aureus* USA 300 clone as the predominant cause of skin and soft-tissue infections. *Ann Intern Med* 2006; 144:309-317.

Klein E, Smith DL, Laxminarayan R. Hospitalizations and deaths caused by methicillin-resistant Staphylococcus aureus, United States, 1999-2005. *Emerg Infect Dis* 2007; 13:1840-1846.

Klevenns RM, Edwards JR, Tenover FC, McDonald LC, Horan T, Gaynes R; National Nosocomial Infections Surveillance System. Changes in epidemiology of methicillin-resistant *Staphylococcus aureus* in intensive care units in US hospitals, 1992-2003. *Clin Infect Dis* 2006;42:389-391.

Klevens RM, Edwards JR, Tenover FC, McDonald LC, Horan T, Gaynes R. Changes in the epidemiology of methicillin-resistant *Staphylococcus aureus* in intensive care units in US hospitals, 1992–2003. *Clin Infect Dis* 2006; 42:389-391.

Kline MD, Humphrey BS, Wang YF, Kourbatova EV, Ray SM, Blumberg HM. Emergence of community-acquired methicillin-resistant *Staphylococcus aureus* USA 300 clone as the predominant cause of skin and soft tissue infections. *Ann Intern Med* 2006;144:309-317.

Kloos WE, Bannerman TL. 1995. Staphylococcus and Micrococcus. In: Murray, P.R., Baron, E.J., Pfaller, M.A., Tenover, F.C., Yolken, R.H. (Eds.), *Manual of Clinical Microbiology,* 6th ed. ASM Press, Washington, D.C., USA, pp. 282-298.

Kluytmans J, van Belkum A, Verbrugh H. Nasal carriage of Staphylococcus aureus: epidemiology, underlying mechanisms, and associated risks. *Clin Microbiol Rev* 1997;10:505-520.

Kluytmans-Vandenbergh MF, Kluytmans JA. Community-acquired methicillin-resistant Staphylococcus aureus: current perspectives. *Clin Microbiol Infect* 2006;12:697-698.

Koga T, Abe T, Inoue H, Takenouchi T, Kitayama A, Yoshida T, Masuda N, Sugihara C, Kakuta M, Nakagawa M, Shibayama T, Matsushita Y, Hirota T, Ohya S, Utsui Y, Fukuoka T, Kuwahara S.. In vitro and in vivo antibacterial activities of CS-023 (RO4908463), a novel parenteral carbapenem. *Antimicrob Agents Chemother* 2005; 49: 3239–3250.

Kollef MH. Inadequate antimicrobial treatment: an important determinant of outcome for hospitalized patients. *Clin Infect Dis* 2000;31:131-138.

Kollef MH. Limitations of vancomycin in the management of resistant staphylococcal infections. *Clin Infect Dis* 2007;45(Suppl 3):S191-195.

Koreen L, Ramaswamy SV, Graviss EA, Naidich S, Musser JM, Kreiswirth BN. spa typing method for discriminating among *Staphylococcus aureus* isolates: implications for use of a single marker to detect genetic micro- and macrovariation. *J Clin Microbiol* 2004;42: 792-799.

Kourbatova EV, Halvosa JS, King MD, Ray SM, White N, Blumberg HM. Emergence of community-associated methicillin-resistant *Staphylococcus aureus* USA300 clone as a cause of healthcare-associated infections among patients with prosthetic joint infections. *Am J Infect Control* 2005;33:385-391.

Kumar A, Roberts D, Wood KE, Light B, Parrillo JE, Sharma S, Suppes R, Feinstein D, Zanotti S, Taiberg L, Gurka D, Kumar A, Cheang M. Duration of hypotension before initiation of effective antimicrobial therapy is the critical determinant of survival in human septic shock. *Crit Care Med* 2006;34:1589-1596.

Labandeira-Rey M, Couzon F, Boisset S, Brown EL, Bes M, Benito Y, Barbu EM, Vazquez V, Höök M, Etienne J, Vandenesch F, Bowden MG. *Staphylococcus aureus* Panton-Valentine leukocidin causes necrotizing pneumonia. *Science* 2007;315:1130-1133.

Lamer C, de Beco V, Soler P, Calvat S, Fagon JY, Dombret MC, Farinotti R, Chastre J, Gibert C. Analysis of vancomycin entry into pulmonary lining fluid by bronchoalveolar lavage in critically ill patients. *Antimicrob Agents Chemother* 1993;37;281-286.

LaPlante KL, Rybak MJ. Clinical glycopeptide-intermediate staphylococci tested against arbekacin, daptomycin, and tigecycline. *Diagn Microbiol Infect Dis* 2004; 50: 125-130.

Leclercq R. Mechanisms of resistance to macrolides and lincosamides: nature of the resistance elements and their clinical implications. *Clin Infect Dis* 2002;34: 482-492.

Lee MC, Rios AM, AtenMF, Mejias A, Cavuoti D, McCracken Jr GH, Hardy RD. Management and outcome of children with skin and soft tissue abscesses caused by community-acquired methicillin-resistant Staphylococcus aureus. *Pediatr Infect Dis J* 2004;23:123-127.

Levine DP, Fromm BS, Reddy BR. Slow response to vancomycin or vancomycin plus rifampin in methicillin-resistant *Staphylococcus aureus* endocarditis. *Ann Intern Med* 1991;115:674-680.

Li JZ, Willke RJ, Rittenhouse BE, Rybak MJ. Effect of linezolid versus vancomycin on length of hospital stay in patients with complicated skin and soft tissue infections caused by known or suspected methicillin-resistant staphylococci: results from a randomized clinical trial. *Surg Infect (Larchmt)* 2003; 4: 57-70.

Lim D, Strynadka NC. Structural basis for the beta lactam resistance of PBP2a from methicillin-resistant *Staphylococcus aureus*. *Nat Struct Biol* 2002; 9: 870–876.

Lina G, Piemont Y, Godail-Gamot F, Bes M, Peter MO, Gauduchon V, Vandenesch F, Etienne J. Involvement of PantoneValentine leukocidin-producing *Staphylococcus aureus* in primary skin infections and pneumonia. *Clin Infect Dis* 1999;29:1128-1132.

Lindsay JA, Holden MT. Understanding the rise of the superbug: investigation of the evolution and genomic variation of *Staphylococcus aureus*. *Funct Integr Genomics* 2006;6: 186-201.

Liu C, Chambers HF. *Staphylococcus aureus* with heterogeneous resistance to vancomycin: epidemiology, clinical significance, and critical assessment of diagnostic methods. *Antimicrob Agents Chemother* 2003; 47: 3040-3045.

Liu C, Graber CJ, Karr M, Diep BA, Basuino L, Schwartz BS, Enright MC, O'Hanlon SJ, Thomas JC, Perdreau-Remington F, Gordon S, Gunthorpe H, Jacobs R, Jensen P, Leoung G, Rumack JS, Chambers HF. A population-based study of the incidence and molecular epidemiology of methicillin-resistant *Staphylococcus aureus* disease in San Francisco, 2004-2005. *Clin Infect Dis* 2008;46(11):1637-1646.

Livermore DM. Can β-lactams be re-engineered to beat MRSA? *Clin Microbiol Infect* 2006;12(Suppl.2):11-16.

Lodise TP Jr, McKinnon PS, Rybak M. Prediction model to identify patients with *Staphylococcus aureus* bacteremia at risk for methicillin-resistance. *Infect Control Hosp Epidemiol* 2003;24:655-671.

LoVecchio F, Perera N, Casanova L, Mulrow M, Pohl A. Board-certified emergency physicians' treatment of skin and soft tissue infections in the community-acquired methicillin-resistant *Staphylococcus aureus* era. *Am J Emerg Med* 2009;27(1):68-70.

Lowy FD, Aiello AE, Bhat M, Johnson-Lawrence VD, Lee MH, Burrell E, Wright LN, Vasquez G, Larson EL. *Staphylococcus aureus* Colonization and Infection in New York State Prisons. *J Infect Dis* 2007; 196:911-918

Lowy FD. *Staphylococcus aureus* infections. N Engl J Med 1998;339:520-532.

Lu D, Holtom P. Community-acquired methicillin-resistant *Staphylococcus aureus*, a new player in sports medicine. *Curr Sports Med Rep* 2005; 4:265-270.

Ma XX, Galiana A, Pedreira W, Mowszowicz M, Christophersen I, Machiavello S, Lope L, Benaderet S, Buela F, Vincentino W, Albini M, Bertaux O, Constenla I, Bagnulo H, Llosa L, Ito T, Hiramatsu K. Community-acquired methicillin-resistant *Staphylococcus aureus*, Uruguay. *Emerg Infect Dis* 2005; 11:973-976.

Maki DG. Control of colonization and transmission of pathogenic bacteria in the hospital. *Ann Intern Med* 1978;89:777-780.

Malachowa N, Sabat A, Gniadkowski M, Krzyszton-Russjan J, Empel J, Miedzobrodzki J, Kosowska-Shick K, Appelbaum PC, Hryniewicz W, 2005. Comparison of multiple-locus variable-number tandem-repeat analysis with pulsed-field gel electrophoresis, spa typing, and multilocus sequence typing for clonal characterization of *Staphylococcus aureus* isolates. *J Clin Microbiol* 2005; 43: 3095-3100.

Mangili A, Bica I, Snydman DR, Hamer DH. Daptomycin-resistant, methicillin-resistant *Staphylococcus aureus* bacteremia. *Clin Infect Dis.* 2005; 40:1058-1060.

Maquelin K, Cookson B, Tassios P, van Belkum A. Current trends in the epidemiological typing of clinically relevant microbes in Europe. *J Microbiol Methods* 2007; 69: 222-226.

Maraha B, van Halteren J, Verzij JM, Wintermans RGF, Buiting AGM. Decolonization of methicillin-resistant *Staphylococcus aureus* using oral vancomycin and topical mupirocin. *Clin Microbiol Infect* 2002; 8: 671-675.

Maree CL, Daum RS, Boyle-Vavra S, Matayoshi K, Miller LG. Community-associated methicillin resistant *Staphylococcus aureus* isolates causing health care-associated infections. *Emerg Infect Dis* 2007;13:236-242.

Markowitz N, Quinn EL, Saravolatz LD. Trimethoprim–sulfamethoxazole compared with vancomycin for the treatment of *Staphylococcus aureus* infection. *Ann Intern Med* 2002; 117:390-398.

Marshall SH, Donskey CJ, Hutton-Thomas R, Salata RA, Rice LB. Gene dosage and linezolid resistance in *Enterococcus faecium* and *Enterococcus faecalis. Antimicrob Agents Chemother* 2002; 46: 3334-3336.

Martinez-Aguilar G, Hammerman WA, Mason Jr EO, Kaplan SL. Clindamycin treatment of invasive infections caused by community acquired, methicillin-resistant and methicillin-susceptible *Staphylococcus aureus* in children. *Pediatr Infect Dis J* 2003; 22:593-598.

Maslow JN, Mulligan ME, Arbeit RD. Molecular epidemiology: application of contemporary techniques to the typing of microorganisms. *Clin Infect Dis* 1993; 17(2): 153-164.

McDougal LK, Steward CD, Killgore GE, Chaitram JM, McAllister SK, Tenover FC. Pulsed-field gel electrophoresis typing of oxacillin-resistant *Staphylococcus aureus* isolates from the United States; establishing a national database. *J Clin Microbiol* 2003;41:5113-5120.

McGinigle K, Gourlay M, Buchanan I. The use of active surveillance cultures in adult intensive care units to reduce methicillin-resistant *Staphylococcus aureus* related morbidity, mortality, and coasts: a systematic review. *Clin Infect Dis* 2008;46:1717-1725.

McHugh CG, Riley LW. Risk factors and costs associated with methicillin-resistant *Staphylococcus aureus* bloodstream infections. *Infect Control Hosp Epidemiol* 2004; 25: 425-430.

Micek ST. Alternatives to vancomycin for the treatment of meticillin resistant *Staphylococcus aureus* infections. *Clin Infect Dis* 2007;45(Suppl 3): S184-190.

Miller LG, Diep AD. Colonization, fomites and virulence: rethinking the pathogenesis of community-associated methicillin-resistant *Staphylococcus aureus* infection. *Clin Infect Dis* 2008;46:752-760.

Miller LG, Perdreau-Remington F, Bayer AS, Diep B, Tan N, Bharadwa K, Tsui J, Perlroth J, Shay A, Tagudar G, Ibebuogu U, Spellberg B. Clinical and epidemiologic characteristics cannot distinguish community-associated methicillin-resistant *Staphylococcus aureus* infection from methicillin-susceptible S. aureus infection: a prospective investigation. *Clin Infect Dis.* 2007;44:471-482.

Minnesota Department of Health. Community-associated methicillin resistant *Staphylococcus aureus* in Minnesota. *Minnesota Department of Heath Disease Control Newsletter* 2004;32:61-72.

Mizen L, Berry V, Woodnutt G. The influence of uptake from the gastrointestinal tract and first-pass effect on oral bioavailability of (Z)-alkyloxyimino penicillins. *J Pharm Pharmacol* 1995; 47: 725–730.

Moellering RC Jr. Current treatment options for community-acquired methicillin resistant *Staphylococcus aureus* infection. *Clin Infect Dis* 2008;46:1032-1037.

Moellering RC Jr. The growing menace of community-acquired methicillin-resistant *Staphylococcus aureus*. *Ann Intern Med* 2006; 144: 368-370.

Moet GJ, Jones RN, Biedenbach DJ, Stilwell MG, Fritsche TR. Contemporary causes of skin and soft tissue infections in North America, Latin America, and Europe: Report from the SENTRY Antimicrobial Surveillance Program (1998–2004). *Diagn Microbiol Infect Dis* 2007; 57: 7-13.

Moise PA, Smyth DS, El Fawal N, Robinson DA, Holden PN, Forrest A, Sakoulas G. Microbiological effects of prior vancomycin use in patients with methicillin-resistant *Staphylococcus aureus* bacteraemia. *J Antimicrob Chemother* 2008; 61: 85-90.

Mongkolrattabithai K, Boyle S, Kahana MD, Daum RS. Severe *Staphylococcus aureus* infections caused by clonally related communityacquired methicillin-susceptible and methicillin-resistant isolates. *Clin Infect Dis* 2003;37:1050-1058.

Montville R, Chen Y, Schaffner DW. Risk assessment of hand washing efficacy using literature and experimental data. *Int J Food Microbiol* 2002;73:305-313.

Moore PC, Lindsay JA. Molecular characterisation of the dominant UK methicillin-resistant *Staphylococcus aureus* strains, EMRSA-15 and EMRSA-16. *J Med Microbiol* 2002;51:516-521.

Moran GJ, Krishnadasan A, Gorwitz RJ, Fosheim GE, McDougal LK, Carey RB, Talan DA; EMERGEncy ID Net Study Group. Methicillin-resistant *S. aureus* infections among patients in the emergency department. *N Engl J Med* 2006; 355:666-674.

Morgan A, Cofer C, Stevens DL. Iclaprim: a novel dihydrofolate reductase inhibitor for skin and soft tissue infections. *Future Microbiol.* 2009;4:131-144.

Mortimer Jr EA, Wolinsky E, Gonzaga AJ, Rammelkamp Jr CH. Role of airborne transmission in staphylococcal infections. *Br Med J* 1996; 1: 319-322.

Mulligan ME, Murray-Leisure KA, Ribner BS, Standiford HC, John JF, Korvick JA, Kauffman CA, Yu VL. Methicillin-resistant *Staphylococcus aureus*: a consensus review of microbiology, pathogenesis, and epidemiology with implications for prevention and management. *Am J Med* 1993; 94: 313-328.

Mutnick AH, Biedenbach DJ, Tunbridge JD, Jones RN. Spectrum and potency evaluation of a new oxazolidinone, linezolid: report from the SENTRY Antimicrobial Surveillance Program, 1998-2000. *Diagn Microbiol Infect* 2002; 43:65-73.

Mwangi MM, Wu SW, Zhou Y, Sieradzki K, de Lencastre H, Richardson P, Bruce D, Rubin E, Myers E, Siggia ED, Tomasz A. Tracking the in vivo evolution of multidrug resistance in *Staphylococcus aureus* by whole-genome sequencing. *Proc Natl Acad Sci U S A* 2007;104:9451-9456.

Nathwani D, Morgan M, Masterton RG, , Dryden M, Cookson BD, French G, Lewis D; British Society for Antimicrobial Chemotherapy Working Party on Community-onset MRSA Infections. Guidelines for UK practice for the diagnosis and management of methicillin resistant *Staphylococcus aureus* (MRSA) infections presenting in the community. *J Antimicrob Chemother* 2008;61:976-994.

Nathwani D. Tygecycline: clinical evidence and formulary positioning. *Int J Antimicrob Agents.* 2005;25:185-192.

National Audit Office. *The management and control of hospital acquired infection in acute NHS trusts in England: report by Controller and Auditor General.* London: Stationery Office; 2000. Paragraphs 15-16.

National Committee for Clinical Laboratory Standards. *Performance standards for antimicrobial susceptibility testing; eighth informational supplement. NCCLS document MS100-SB.* Wayne, PA: National Committee for Clinical Laboratory Standards, 1998.

Noda M, Kato I. Purification and crystallization of staphylococcal leukocidin. *Methods Enzymol* 1988; 165: 22-32.

Nomura S, Hanaki H, Unemi N. In vitro antibacterial activity of TOC-50, a new parenteral cephalosporin against methicillin-resistant *Staphylococcus aureus* and Staphylococcus epidermidis. *Chemotherapy* 1996; 42: 253–258.

Norden CW, Shaffer M. Treatment of experimental chronic osteomyelitis due to *Staphylococcus aureus* with vancomycin and rifampin.*J Infect Dis.* 1983;147(2):352-357.

O'Hanlon SJ, Enright MC. A novel bactericidal fabric coating with potent in vitro activity against meticillin-resistant *Staphylococcus aureus* (MRSA). *Int J Antimicrob Agents* 2009;33(5):427-431.

Oie S, Kamiya A. Survival of methicillin-resistant *Staphylococcus aureus* (MRSA) on naturally contaminated dry mops. *J Hosp Infect* 1996;34: 145-149.

Okuma K, Iwakawa K, Turnidge JD, Grubb WB, Bell JM, O'Brien FG, Coombs GW, Pearman JW, Tenover FC, Kapi M, Tiensasitorn C, Ito T, Hiramatsu K. Dissemination of new methicillin-resistant *Staphylococcus aureus* clones in the community. *J Clin Microbiol* 2002;40:4289-4294.

Olive DM, Bean P. Principles and applications of methods for DNA-based typing of microbial organisms. *J Clin Microbiol* 1999; 37: 1661-1669.

Oliveira DC, Milheirico C, de Lencastre H. Redefining a structural variant of staphylococcal cassette chromosome *mec*, SCCmec type VI. *Antimicrob Agents Chemother* 2006; 50: 3457-3459.

Padmanabhan RA, Fraser TG. The emergence of methicillin-resistant *Staphylococcus aureus* in the community. *Cleve Clin J Med* 2005; 72:235–241.

Pan ES, Diep BA, Charlebois ED, Auerswald C, Carleton HA, Sensabaugh GF, Perdreau-Remington F. Population dynamics of nasal strains of methicillin-resistant *Staphylococcus aureus*-and their relation to community-associated disease activity. *J Infect Dis* 2005;192:811-818.

Pankey GA. Tigecycline. *J Antimicrob Chemother*. 2005;56:470-480.

Panton PN, Valentine FCO. Staphylococcal toxin. Lancet 1932; 222: 506-508.

Parras F, Del Carmen Guerrero M, Bouza E, Blazquez MJ, Moreno S, Menarguez MC, Cercenado E. Comparative study of mupirocin and oral cotrimoxazole plus topical fusidic acid in eradication of nasal carriage of methicillin-resistant *Staphylococcus aureus*. *Antimicrob Agents Chemother* 1995; 39: 175-179.

Patel JB, Jevitt LA, Hageman J, McDonald LC, Tenover FC. An association between reduced susceptibility to daptomycin and reduced susceptibility to vancomycin in *Staphylococcus aureus*. *Clin Infect Dis* 2006; 42: 1652-1653.

Paterson DL. Clinical experience with recently approved antibiotics. *Cur Op Pharmacol*. 2006;6:486-490.

Peleg AY, Munckhof WJ, Kleinschmidt SL, Stephens AJ, Huygens F. Life-threatening community-acquired methicillin-resistant *Staphylococcus aureus* infection in Australia. *Eur J Clin Microbiol Infect Dis* 2005; 24:384-387.

Perl TM, Cullen JJ, Wenzel RP. Intranasal mupirocin to prevent postoperative *Staphylococcus aureus* infections. *N Engl J Med* 2002;346:1871-1877.

Peters MJ, Sarria JC. Clinical characteristics of linezolid-resistant *Staphylococcus aureus* infections. *Am J Med Sci.* 2005;330:102-104.

Petersen PJ, Bradford PA, Weiss WJ, Murphy TM, Sum PE, Projan SJ. In vitro and in vivo activities of tigecycline (GAR-936), daptomycin, and comparative antimicrobial agents against glycopeptide-intermediate *Staphylococcus aureus* and other resistant gram-positive pathogens. *Antimicrob Agents Chemother* 2002;46:2595–2601.

Peterson LR, Quick JN, Jensen B, Homann S, Johnson S, Tenquist J, Shanholtzer C, Petzel RA, Sinn L, Gerding DN. Emergence of ciprofloxacin resistance in nosocomial methicillin resistant *Staphylococcus aureus* isolates. *Arch Intern Med* 1990; 150: 2151-2155.

Pittet D, Hugonnet S, Harbarth S, Mourouga P, Sauvan V, Touveneau S, Perneger TV Effectiveness of a hospital-wide program to improve compliance with hand hygiene. *Lancet* 2000;356:1307-1312.

Pope SD, Roecker AM. Vancomycin for treatment of invasive, multi-drug resistant *Staphylococcus aureus* infections. *Expert Opin Pharmacother* 2007; 8: 1245-1261.

Proctor RA. Role of folate antagonists in the treatment of methicillin-resistant *Staphylococcus aureus* infection. *Clin Infect Dis.* 2008; 46(4):584-593.

Purcell K, Fergie J. Epidemic of community-acquired methicillin resistant *Staphylococcus aureus* infections: a 14-year study at Driscoll Children's Hospital. *Arch Pediatr Adolesc Med* 2005; 159:980-985.

Raimundo O, Heussler H, Bruhn JB, Suntrarachun S, Kelly Deighton MA, Garland SM. Molecular epidemiology of coagulase negative staphylococcal bacteramia in a newborn intensive care unit. *J Hosp Infect* 2002; 51: 33-42.

Reagan DR, Doebbeling BN, Pfaller MA, Sheetz CT, Houston AK, Hollis RJ, Wenzel RP. Elimination of coincident *Staphylococcus aureus* nasal and hand carriage with intranasal application of mupirocin calcium ointment. *Ann Intern Med* 1991;114:101-106.

Rehm SJ, Boucher H, Levine D, Campion M, Eisenstein BI, Vigliani GA, Corey GR, Abrutyn E. Daptomycin versus vancomycin plus gentamicin for treatment of bacteraemia and endocarditis due to *Staphylococcus aureus*: subset analysis of patients infected with methicillin-resistant isolates. *J Antimicrob Chemother.* 2008 Dec;62(6):1413-1421.

Ribeiro A, Dias C, Silva-Carvalho MC, Berquó L, Ferreira FA, Santos RN, Ferreira-Carvalho BT, Figueiredo AM. First report of infection with community-acquired methicillin-resistant *Staphylococcus aureus* in South America. *J Clin Microbiol* 2005; 43:1985-1988.

Rice LB. Do we really need new anti-infective drugs? *Curr Opin Pharmacol* 2003;3:459-463.

Rihn JA, Posfay-Barbe K, Harner CD, Macurak A, Farley A, Greenawalt K, Michaels MG. Community-acquired methicillin-resistant *Staphylococcus aureus* outbreak in a local high school football team: unsuccessful interventions. *Pediatr Infect Dis J* 2005; 24:841-843.

Robinson DA, Enright MC. Multilocus sequence typing and the evolution of methicillin-resistant *Staphylococcus aureus*. *Clin Microbiol Infect* 2004; 10: 92-97.

Robinson DA, Kearns AM, Holmes A, Morrison D, Grundmann H, Edwards G, O'Brien FG, Tenover FC, McDougal LK, Monk AB, Enright MC. Re-emergence of early pandemic *Staphylococcus aureus* as a community-acquired methicillin-resistant clone. *Lancet* 2005; 365:1256-1258.

Rodloff AC , Leclercq R, Debbia EA, Cantón R , Oppenheim BA, Dowzicky MJ. Comparative analysis of antimicrobial susceptibility among organisms from France, Germany, Italy, Spain and the UK as part of the tigecycline evaluation and surveillance trial. 1: *Clin Microbiol Infect.* 2008;14(4):307-314.

Rollason J, Bastin L, Hilton AC, Pillay DG, Worthington T, McKeon C, Dec P, Burrows K, Lambert PA. Epidemiology of community-acquired methicillin resistant *Staphylococcus aureus* obtained from the UK West Midlands region. *J Hosp Infect* 2008; 70(4):314-320.

Rose WE, Leonard SN, Sakoulas G, Kaatz GW, Zervos MJ, Sheth A, Carpenter CF, Rybak MJ. Daptomycin activity against *Staphylococcus aureus* following vancomycin exposure in an in vitro pharmacodynamic model with simulated endocardial vegetations. *Antimicrob Agents Chemother* 2008;52:831-836.

Rosenthal A, White D, Churilla S, Brodie S, Katz KC. Optimal surveillance culture sites for detection of methicillin-resistant *Staphylococcus aureus* in newborns. *J Clin Microbiol* 2006;44:4234-4236.

Rossney A, Morgan P, O'Connell B. Community-acquired PVL+MRSA in Ireland: a preliminary report. *Euro Surveill* 2005; 10(4):E050421.1.

Rouse MS, Steckelberg JM, Patel R. In vitro activity of ceftobiprole, daptomycin, linezolid, and vancomycin against methicillin-resistant staphylococci associated with endocarditis and bone and joint infection. *Diagn Microbiol Infect Dis* 2007;58:363–365.

Rubinstein E, Bompart F. Activity of quinupristin/dalfopristin against gram-positive bacteria: clinical applications and therapeutic potential. *J Antimicrob Chemother:* 1997;39(Suppl A):139-143.

Ruhe JJ, Menon A. Tetracyclines as an oral treatment option for patients with community onset skin and soft tissue infections caused by methicillin-resistant *Staphylococcus aureus. Antimicrob Agents Chemother 2007;* 51:3298-3303.

Ruhe JJ, Monson T, Bradsher RW, Menon A. Use of long-acting tetracyclines for methicillin-resistant *Staphylococcus aureus* infections: case series and review of the literature. *Clin Infect Dis* 2005; 40: 1429-1434.

Ruhe JJ, Smith N, Bradsher RW, Menon A. Community-onset methicillin-resistant *Staphylococcus aureus* skin and soft-tissue infections: impact of antimicrobial therapy on outcome. *Clin Infect Dis* 2007; 44: 777-784.

Rybak MJ. The pharmacokinetic and pharmacodynamic properties of vancomycin. *Clin Infect Dis* 2006;42(Suppl 1):S35-39.

Sader HS, Fritsche TR, Jones RN. Antimicrobial activity of daptomycin and selected comparators tested against bloodstream *Staphylococcus aureus* isolates from hemodialysis patients. *Int J Infect Dis* 2009; 13, 291-295

Sader HS, Fritsche TR, Jones RN. Daptomycin bactericidal activity and correlation between disk and broth microdilution method results in testing of *Staphylococcus aureus* strains with decreased susceptibility to vancomycin. *Antimicrob Agents Chemother* 2006; 50(7):2330-2336.

Saiman L, O'Keefe M, Graham PL. Hospital transmission of community acquired methicillin-resistant *Staphylococcus aureus* among postpartum women. *Clin Infect Dis* 2003;37:1313-1319.

Sakoulas G, Moellering RC Jr. Increasing antibiotics resistance among methicillin resistant *Staphylococcus aureus* strains. *Clin Infect Dis* 2008;46:S360-S367.

Sakoulas G, Moellering RC, Jr., Eliopoulos GM. Adaptation of methicillin-resistant *Staphylococcus aureus* in the face of vancomycin therapy. *Clin Infect Dis* 2006; 42 Suppl 1: S40-S50.

Salgado CD, Farr BM, Calfee DP. Community-acquired methicillin-resistant Staphylococcus aureus: a meta-analysis of prevalence and risk factors. *Clin Infect Dis* 2003; 36:131-139.

Sancak B, Ercis S, Menemenlioglu D, Colakoglu S, Hascelik G. Methicillin-resistant *Staphylococcus aureus* heterogeneously resistant to vancomycin in a Turkish university hospital. *J Antimicrob Chemother* 2005; 56: 519-523.

Saravolatx LD, Markowitz N, Arking L, Pohlod D, Fisher E. Methicillin-resistant *Staphylococcus aureus*: epidemiologic observations during a community acquired outbreak. *Ann Intern Med* 1982;96(1):11-16.

Saulnier P, Bourneix C, Prevost G, Andremont A. Random amplified polymorphic DNA assay is less discriminant than pulsed-field gel electrophoresis for typing strains of methicillin-resistant *Staphylococcus aureus*, *J Clin Microbiol* 1993; 31: 982-985.

Schneider P, Hawser S, Islam K. Iclaprim, a novel diaminopyrimidine with potent activity on trimethoprim sensitive and resistant bacteria. *Bioorg Med Chem Lett* 2003;13:4217-1421.

Schneider-Lindner VA, Delaney JA, Dial S, Dascal A, Suissa S. Antimicrobial drugs and community-acquired methicillin-resistant *Staphylococcus aureus*, United Kingdom. *Emerg Infect Dis* 2007;13:994-1000.

Schulz P, Allen M, Murray Q, Smith SA, Goss L, Carrico R, Ramirez J. Infections due to community acquired methicillin-resistant *Staphylococcus aureus*: an emergent epidemic in Kentucky. *J Ky Med Assoc* 2005; 103:194-203.

Seybold U, Kourbatova EV, Johnson JG, Halvosa SJ, Wang YF, King MD, Ray SM, Blumberg HM. Emergence of community associated methicillin-resistant *Staphylococcus aureus* USA300 genotype as a major cause of health-care associated blood stream infections. *Clin Infect Dis* 2006;42:647-656.

Shastry L, Rahimian J, Lascher S. Community-associated methicillin-resistant *Staphylococcus aureus* skin and soft tissue infections in men who have sex with men in New York City. *Arch Intern Med* 2007;167:854-857.

Shinefield H, Black S, Fattom A, Horwith G, Rasgon S, Ordonez J, Yeoh H, Law D, Robbins JB, Schneerson R, Muenz L, Fuller S, Johnson J, Fireman B, Alcorn H, Naso R. Use of a *Staphylococcus aureus* conjugate vaccine in patients receiving hemodialysis. *N Engl J Med* 2002;346:491-496.

Shiomori T, Miyamoto H, Makishima K, Yoshida M, Fujiyoshi T, Udaka T, Inaba T, Hiraki N. Evaluation of bedmaking-related airborne and surface methicillin-resistant *Staphylococcus aureus* contamination. *J Hosp Infect* 2002; 50: 30-35.

Shitrit P, Gottesman BS, Katzir M, Kilman A, Ben-Nissan Y, Chowers M. Active surveillance for methicillin resistant *Staphylococcus aureus* (MRSA) decreases the incidence of MRSA bacteremia. *Infect Control Hosp Epidemiol* 2006;27:1004-1008.

Shopsin B, Gomez M, Montgomery SO, Smith DH, Waddington M, Dodge DE, Bost DA, Riehman M, Naidich S, Kreiswirth BN. Evaluation of protein A gene polymorphic region DNA sequencing for typing of *Staphylococcus aureus* strains. *J Clin Microbiol* 1999; 37: 3556-3563.

Shore A, Rossney AS, Keane CT, Enright MC, Coleman DC. Seven novel variants of the staphylococcal chromosomal cassette mec in methicillin-resistant *Staphylococcus aureus* isolates from Ireland. *Antimicrob Agents Chemother* 2005; 49: 2070-2083.

Siberry GK, Tekle T, Carroll K, Dick J. Failure of clindamycin treatment of methicillin-resistant *Staphylococcus aureus* expressing inducible clindamycin resistance in vitro. *Clin Infect Dis* 2003;37:1257-1260.

Siegel JD, Rhinehart E, Jackson M, Chiarello L; Healthcare Infection Control Practices Advisory Committee. Management of multidrug-resistant organisms in healthcare settings, 2006. *Am J Infect Control* 2007;35(10 Suppl 2):S165-193.

Siegman-Igra Y, Reich P, Orni-Wasserlauf R, Schwartz D, Giladi M. The role of vancomycin in the persistence or recurrence of *Staphylococcus aureus* bacteraemia. *Scandinavian Journal of Infectious Diseases* 2005;37(8):572-578.

Sievert DM, Rudrik JT, Patel JP, McDonald LC, Wilkins MJ, Hageman JC. Vancomycin-resistant *Staphylococcus aureus* in the United States, 2002-2006. *Clin Infect Dis* 2008;46:668-674.

Solberg CO. Spread of *Staphylococcus aureus* in hospitals: causes and prevention. *Scand. J Infect Dis* 2000;32: 587-595.

spectrum antibiotic for the treatment of multi-resistant and other gram-positive pathogens. *Clin Microbial Newsl.* 1999;21:103-112.

Spellberg B, Powers JH, Brass EP, Miller LG, Edwards JE Jr. Trends in antimicrobial drug development: implications for the future. *Clin Infect Dis.* 2004;38:1279-1286.

Steinberg JP, Clark CC, Hackman BO. Nosocomial and community-acquired *Staphylococcus aureus* bacteremias from 1980 to 1993: impact of intravascular devices and methicillin resistance. *Clin Infect Dis* 1996;23(2):255-259.

Steinkraus G, White R, Friedrich L. Vancomycin MIC creep in nonvancomycin-intermediate *Staphylococcus aureus* (VISA), vancomycin-susceptible clinical methicillin-resistant S. aureus (MRSA) blood isolates from 2001–05. *J Antimicrob Chemother* 2007; 60: 788-794.

Stevens DL, Bisno AL, Chambers HF, Everett ED, Dellinger P, Goldstein EJ, Gorbach SL, Hirschmann JV, Kaplan EL, Montoya JG, Wade JC. Practice guidelines for the diagnosis and management of skin and soft-tissue infections. *Clin Infect Dis* 2005; 41:1373-1406.

Stevens DL, Herr D, Lampiris H, Hunt JL, Batts DH, Hafkin B. Linezolid versus vancomycin for the treatment of methicillin-resistant *Staphylococcus aureus* infections. Clin Infect Dis 2002; 34: 1481-1490.

Stevens DL. The role of vancomycin in the treatment paradigm. *Clin Infect Dis* 2006; 42(Suppl 1):S51-57.

Stevenson KB, Searle K, Stoddard GJ, Samore M. Methicillin-resistant *Staphylococcus aureus* and vancomycin-resistant enterococci in rural communities, western United States. *Emerg Infect Dis* 2005; 11:895–903.

Stryjewski ME, Chu VH, O'Riordan WD, Warren BL, Dunbar LM, Young DM, Vallée M, Fowler VG Jr, Morganroth J, Barriere SL, Kitt MM, Corey GR; FAST 2 Investigator Group. Telavancin versus standard therapy for treatment of complicated skin and skin structure infections caused by Gram-positive bacteria: FAST 2 study. *Antimicrob Agents Chemother* 2006;50:862-867.

Stryjewski ME, Szczech LA, Benjamin DK, Jr., Inrig JK, Kanafani ZA, Engemann JJ, Chu VH, Joyce MJ, Reller LB, Corey GR, Fowler VG, Jr. Use of vancomycin or first-generation cephalosporins for the treatment of hemodialysis-dependent patients with methicillin susceptible *Staphylococcus aureus* bacteremia. *Clin Infect Dis* 2007; 44 (2): 190-196.

Styers D, Sheehan DJ, Hogan P, Sahm DF. Laboratory-based surveillance of current antimicrobial resistance patterns and trends among *Staphylococcus aureus*: 2005 status in the United States. *Ann Clin Microbiol Antimicrob* 2006;5:2.

Suggs AH, Maranan MC, Boyle-Vavra S, Daum RS. Methicillin-resistant and borderline methicillin-resistant asymptomatic *Staphylococcus aureus* colonization in children without identifiable risk factors. *Pediatr Infect Dis J.* 1999;18:410-414.

Sundelof JG, Thompson R, White KM, Sasor MW, Cama L, Kropp H. Pharmacokinetics in nonhuman primates of a prototype carbapenem active against methicillin-resistant *Staphylococcus aureus*. *Antimicrob Agents Chemother* 1996; 40: 795–798.

Takano T, Higuchi W, Otsuka T, Baranovich T, Enany S, Saito K, Isobe H, Dohmae S, Ozaki K, Takano M, Iwao Y, Shibuya M, Okubo T, Yabe S, Shi D, Reva I, Teng LJ, Yamamoto T. Novel characteristics of community-acquired methicillin-resistant *Staphylococcus aureus* belonging to multilocus sequence type 59 in Taiwan. *Antimicrob Agents Chemother* 2008; 52: 837-845.

Tambic A, Power EGM, Tambic T, Snur I, French GL. Epidemiological analysis of meticillin-resistant *Staphylococcus aureus* in a Zagreb trauma hospital using a randomly amplified polymorphic DNA-typing method. *Eur J Microbiol Infect Dis* 1999;18:335-340.

Tang YW, Procop GW, Persing DH. Molecular diagnostics of infectious diseases. *Clin Chem* 1997;43:2021-2038.

Tenover FC, Arbeit RD, Goering RV, Mickelsen PA, Murray BE, Persing DH, Swaminathan B. Interpreting chromosomal DNA restriction patterns produced by pulsed-field gel electrophoresis: criteria for bacterial strain typing. *J Clin Microbiol* 1995; 33: 2233-2239.

Tenover FC, McDougal LK, Goering RV, Killgore G, Projan SJ, Patel JB, Dunman PM. Characterization of a strain of community-associated methicillin-resistant *Staphylococcus aureus* widely disseminated in the United States. *J Clin Microbiol* 2006;44:108-118.

Tenover FC, Moellering Jr RC. The rationale for revising the Clinical and Laboratory Standards Institute vancomycin minimal inhibitory concentration interpretive criteria for Staphylococcus aureus. *Clinical Infectious Diseases* 2007 May 1;44(9):1208-1215.

Thal LA, Zervos MJ. Occurrence and epidemiology of resistance to virginiamycin and streptogramins. *J Antimicrob Chemother* 1999;43: 171-176.

Tiemersma EW, Bronzwaer SL, Lyytikainen O, Degener JE, Schrijnemakers P, Bruinsma N, Monen J, Witte W, Grundman H. Methicillin resistant *Staphylococcus aureus* in Europe, 1999–2002. *Emerg Infect Dis* 2004; 10: 1627-1634.

Torell E, Molin D, Tano E, Ehrenborg C, Ryden C. Community-acquired pneumonia and bacteraemia in a healthy young woman caused by methicillin resistant *Staphylococcus aureus* (MRSA) carrying the genes encoding Panton–Valentine leukocidin (PVL). *Scand J Infect Dis* 2005; 37: 902-904.

Tristan A, Bes M, Meugnier H, Lina G, Bozdogan B, Courvalin P, Reverdy ME, Enright MC, Vandenesch F, Etienne J. Global distribution of Panton-Valentine leukocidin-positive methicillin-resistant *Staphylococcus aureus*, 2006. *Emerg Infect Dis* 2007; 13: 594-600.

Tsiodras S, Gold HS, Sakoulas G, Eliopoulos GM, Wennersten C, Venkataraman L, Moellering RC, Ferraro MJ. Linezolid resistance in a clinical isolate of *Staphylococcus aureus*. *Lancet* 2001; 358: 207-208.

Turabelidze G, Lin M, Wolkoff B, Dodson D, Gladbach S, Zhu BP. Personal hygiene and methicillin-resistant *Staphylococcus aureus* infection. *Emerg Infect Dis* 2004;10:941-944.

U.S. Congress, Office of Technology Assessment. Impacts of antibiotic-resistant bacteria. Washington, DC: US Government Printing Office; September 1995.

Valls V, Gomez-Herruz P, Gonzalez-Palacios R, Cuadros JA, Romanyk JP, Ena J. Long-term efficacy of a program to control methicillin-resistant *Staphylococcus aureus. Eur J Clin Microbiol Infect Dis* 1994; 13: 90-95.

Vandenesch F, Naimi T, Enright MC, Lina G, Nimmo GR, Heffernan H, Liassine N, Bes M, Greenland T, Reverdy ME, Etienne J. Community-acquired methicillin-resistant *Staphylococcus aureus* carrying Panton-Valentine leukocidin genes: worldwide emergence. *Emerg Infect Dis* 2003; 9:978-984.

Vergidis PI, Falagas ME. New antibiotic agents for bloodstream infections. *International Journal of Antimicrobial Agents* 32S (2008) S60–S65.

Vidal PM, Trindade PA, Garcia TO, Pacheco RL, Costa SF, Reinert C, Hiramatsu K, Mamizuka EM, Garcia CP, Levin AS. Differences between "classical" risk factors for infections caused by methicillin-resistant *Staphylococcus aureus* (MRSA) and risk factors for nosocomial bloodstream infections caused by multiple clones of the staphylococcal cassette chromosome mec type IV MRSA strain. *Infect Control Hosp Epidemiol* 2009;30(2):139-145.

Vikram HR, Havill NL, Koeth LM, Boyce JM. Clinical progression of methicillin-resistant *Staphylococcus aureus* vertebral osteomyelitis associated with reduced susceptibility to daptomycin. *J Clin Microbiol.* 2005;43: 5384-5387.

von Eiff C, Becker K, Machka K, Stammer H, Peters G. Nasal carriage as a source of *Staphylococcus aureus* bacteremia. Study group. *N Engl J Med* 2001;344:11-16.

Voyich JM, Otto M, Mathema B, Braughton KR, Whitney AR, Welty D, Long RD, Dorward DW, Gardner DJ, Lina G, Kreiswirth BN, DeLeo FR. Is Panton-Valentine Leukocidin the major virulence determinant in community-associated methicillin resistant *Staphylococcus aureus* disease? *J Infect Dis* 2006;194:1761-1770.

Wagenvoort JH, Sluijsmans W, Penders RJ. Better environmental survival of outbreak vs. sporadic MRSA isolates. *J Hosp Infect* 2000; 45: 231-234.

Walsh TJ, Standiford HC, Reboli AC, John JF, Mulligan ME, Ribner BS, Montgomerie JZ, Goetz MB, Mayhall CG, Rimland D. Randomized double-blinded trial of rifampin with either novobiocin or trimethoprim–sulfamethoxazole against methicillin-resistant *Staphylococcus aureus* colonization: prevention of antimicrobial resistance and effect of host factors on outcome. *Antimicrob Agents Chemother* 1993; 37: 1334-1342.

Walsh TR, Howe RA. The prevalence and mechanisms of vancomycin resistance in *Staphylococcus aureus*. *Ann Rev Microbiol* 2002; 56: 657-675.

Wang R, Braughton KR, Kretschmer D, Bach TH, Queck SY, Li M, Kennedy AD, Dorward DW, Klebanoff SJ, Peschel A, DeLeo FR, Otto M. Identificaiton of novel cytolytic peptides as key virulence determinants for community-associated MRSA. *Nat Med* 2007;13:1510-1514.

Warren DK, Liao RS, Merz LR, Eveland M, Dunne Jr WM. Detection of methicillin-resistant *Staphylococcus aureus* directly from nasal swab specimens by a real-time PCR assay. *J Clin Microbiol* 2004;42:5578-5581.

Weathers L, Riggs D, Santeiro M, Weibley RE. Aerosolized vancomycin for treatment of airway colonization by methicillin-resistant *Staphylococcus aureus*. *Pediatr Infect Dis J* 1990; 9: 220-221.

Weber JT. Community-associated methicillin-resistant *Staphylococcus aureus*. *Clin Infect Dis* 2005; 41(Suppl 4):S269-S272.

Weigelt J, Itani K, Stevens D, Lau W, Dryden M, Knirsch C. Linezolid versus vancomycin in treatment of complicated skin and soft tissue infections. *Antimicrob Agents Chemother* 2005; 49: 2260-2266.

Wenzel RP. The antibiotic pipeline challenges, costs, and values. *N Engl J Med* 2004;351:523-526.

Whitby M, McLaws ML, Berry G. Risk of death from methicillin resistant *Staphylococcus aureus* bacteraemia: a meta-analysis. *Med J Aust* 2001; 175: 264-267.

Witt Rt, Kanhai V, vanLeeuwen WB. Comparison of theDiversiLab™system, Pulsed-Field Gel Electrophoresis and Multi-Locus Sequence Typing for the characterization of epidemic reference MRSA strains. *J Microbiol Methods* 2009; 77: 130-133.

Woodin AM. Purification of the two components of leucocidin fron *Staphylococcus aureus*. *Biochem J* 1960; 75:158-165.

Wootton M, MacGowan AP, Walsh TR. Comparative bactericidal activities of daptomycin and vancomycin against glycopeptides intermediate *Staphylococcus aureus* (GISA) and heterogeneous GISA isolates. *Antimicrob Agents Chemother* 2006; 50: 4195-4197.

Wu SW, de Lencastre H, Tomasz A. Recruitment of the mecA gene homologue of Staphylococcus sciuri into a resistance determinant and expression of the resistant phenotype in *Staphylococcus aureus*. *J Bacteriol* 2001; 183: 2417-2424.

Wunderink RG, Rello J, Cammarata SK, Croos-Dabrera RV, Kollef MH. Linezolid vs vancomycin: analysis of two double-blind studies of patients with methicillin-resistant *Staphylococcus aureus* nosocomial pneumonia. *Chest* 2003; 124: 1789–1797.

Yamasaki O, Kaneko J, Morizane S, Akiyama H, Arata J, Narita S, Chiba J, Kamio Y, Iwatsuki K. The association between *Staphylococcus aureus* strains carrying Panton-Valentine leukocidin genes and the development of deep-seated follicular infection. *Clin Infect Dis* 2005;40:381-385.

Yang ES, Tan J, Rieg G, et al. Body site colonization prevalence in patients with community-associated methicillin-resistant *Staphylococcus aureus* infections [abstract 285]. In: Program and Abstracts of the 45th Annual *Meeting of the Infectious Diseases Society of America* (San Diego). Alexandria, VA: Infectious Diseases Society of America, 2007;107.

Yilmaz G, Aydin K, Iskender S, Caylan R, Koksal I. Detection and prevalence of inducible clindamycin resistance in staphylococci. *J Med Microbiol* 2007; 56, 342-345.

Yin LY, Lazzarini L, Li F, Stevens CM, Calhoun JH. Comparative evaluation of tigecycline and vancomycin, with and without rifampicin, in the treatment of methicillin-resistant *Staphylococcus aureus* experimental osteomyelitis in a rabbit model. *J Antimicrob Chemother.* 2005; 55(6):995-1002.

Yuk JH, Dignani MC, Harris RL, Bradshaw MW, Williams Jr TW. Minocycline as an alternative antistaphylococcal agent. *Rev Infect Dis* 1991; 13:1023-1024.

Zinderman CE, Conner B, Malakooti MA, LaMar JE, Armstrong A, Bohnker BK. Community-acquired methicillin-resistant *Staphylococcus aureus* among military recruits. *Emerg Infect Dis* 2004;10:941-944.

INDEX

D

E